HISTORY OF THE AVON LONGITUDINAL STUDY OF PARENTS AND CHILDREN (ALSPAC), c.1980–2000

The transcript of a Witness Seminar held by the History of Modern Biomedicine Research Group, Queen Mary, University of London, on 24 May 2011

Edited by C Overy, L A Reynolds and E M Tansey

Volume 44   2012

First published by Queen Mary, University of London, 2012

The History of Modern Biomedicine Research Group is funded by the Wellcome Trust, which is a registered charity, no. 210183.

ISBN 9780 90223 878 7

All volumes are freely available online at www.history.qmul.ac.uk/research/modbiomed/ wellcome_witnesses/

Please cite as: Overy C, Reynolds L A, Tansey E M. (eds) (2012) *History of the Avon Longitudinal Study of Parents and Children (ALSPAC), c.1980–2000*. Wellcome Witnesses to Twentieth Century Medicine, vol. 44. London: Queen Mary, University of London.

CONTENTS

ILLUSTRATIONS AND CREDITS

ABBREVIATIONS

ABRC	Advisory Board for the Research Councils
ALSPAC	Avon Longitudinal Study of Pregnancy and Childhood / Parents and Children
ARC	Asthma Research Council
BBSRC	Biotechnology and Biological Sciences Research Council
BCS70	1970 British Cohort Study
BIS	Business Innovation and Skills
BPA	British Paediatric Association
DoH	Department of Health
EBV	Epstein-Barr Virus
EDTA	Ethylenediaminetetraacetic acid
ELSPAC	European Longitudinal Study of Pregnancy and Childhood
EMLA	Eutectic Mixture of Local Anesthetics
ESDS	Economic and Social Data Service
ESRC	Economic and Social Research Council
GWAS	Genome-wide association study
HPA	Health Protection Agency
LREC	Local research ethics committee
MCS	Millennium Cohort Study
MRC	Medical Research Council
NCDS	National Child Development Study
NCT	National Childbirth Trust
NFIP	National Foundation for Infantile Paralysis
NIH	National Institutes of Health

NRES	National Research Ethics Service
NSHD	National Survey of Health & Development
PCR	Polymerase chain reaction
PHLS	Public Health Laboratory Service
TAP	Teenage Advisory Panel
UBHT	United Bristol Healthcare Trust
WHO	World Health Organization

WITNESS SEMINARS:
MEETINGS AND PUBLICATIONS [1]

In 1990 the Wellcome Trust created a History of Twentieth Century Medicine Group, associated with the Academic Unit of the Wellcome Institute for the History of Medicine, to bring together clinicians, scientists, historians and others interested in contemporary medical history. Among a number of other initiatives the format of Witness Seminars, used by the Institute of Contemporary British History to address issues of recent political history, was adopted, to promote interaction between these different groups, to emphasize the potential benefits of working jointly, and to encourage the creation and deposit of archival sources for present and future use. In June 1999 the Governors of the Wellcome Trust decided that it would be appropriate for the Academic Unit to enjoy a more formal academic affiliation and turned the Unit into the Wellcome Trust Centre for the History of Medicine at UCL from 1 October 2000 to 30 September 2010. The History of Twentieth Century Medicine Group has been part of the School of History, Queen Mary, University of London, since October 2010, as the History of Modern Biomedicine Research Group, which the Wellcome Trust continues to fund.

The Witness Seminar is a particularly specialized form of oral history, where several people associated with a particular set of circumstances or events are invited to come together to discuss, debate, and agree or disagree about their memories. To date, the History of Twentieth Century Medicine Group has held more than 50 meetings, most of which have been published, as listed on pages pages xiii–xvii.

Subjects are usually proposed by, or through, members of the Programme Committee of the Group, which includes professional historians of medicine, practising scientists and clinicians, and once an appropriate topic has been agreed, suitable participants are identified and invited. This inevitably leads to further contacts, and more suggestions of people to invite. As the organization of the meeting progresses, a flexible outline plan for the meeting is devised, usually with assistance from the meeting's chairman, and some participants are invited to 'set the ball rolling' on particular themes, by speaking for a short period to initiate and stimulate further discussion.

---

[1] The following text also appears in the 'Introduction' to recent volumes of *Wellcome Witnesses to Twentieth Century Medicine* as listed on pages xiii–xvii.

Each meeting is fully recorded, the tapes are transcribed and the unedited transcript is immediately sent to every participant. Each is asked to check his or her own contributions and to provide brief biographical details. The editors turn the transcript into readable text, and participants' minor corrections and comments are incorporated into that text, while biographical and bibliographical details are added as footnotes, as are more substantial comments and additional material provided by participants. The final scripts are then sent to every contributor, accompanied by forms assigning copyright to the Wellcome Trust. Copies of all additional correspondence received during the editorial process are deposited with the records of each meeting in archives and manuscripts, Wellcome Library, London.

As with all our meetings, we hope that even if the precise details of some of the technical sections are not clear to the non-specialist, the sense and significance of the events will be understandable. Our aim is for the volumes that emerge from these meetings to inform those with a general interest in the history of modern medicine and medical science; to provide historians with new insights, fresh material for study, and further themes for research; and to emphasize to the participants that events of the recent past, of their own working lives, are of proper and necessary concern to historians.

ACKNOWLEDGEMENTS

Professor Jean Golding and Professor Marcus Pembrey suggested 'The History of the Avon Longitudinal Study of Parents and Children' as a suitable topic for a Witness Seminar and helped us to plan the meeting, for which we are grateful. We also thank Professor Catherine Peckham for her excellent chairing of the occasion, Professor David Gordon for writing the introduction to these published proceedings, and Dr Alan Doyle who, unable to attend the meeting, read and commented on a draft transcript. We are grateful to Mrs Yasmin Iles-Caven, Mrs Ruth Bowles and Professor Marcus Pembrey for providing illustrations. For permission to reproduce images included here we thank Professor Jean Golding, Mrs Bowles and the *Bristol Evening Post*; material is also reproduced under the Open Parliament Licence.

To ensure the smooth running of all our meetings, we depend a great deal on Wellcome Trust staff: the Audiovisual Department, Catering, Reception, Security and Wellcome Images. We thank Mr Akio Morishima who supervised the design and production of this volume, our indexer Ms Liza Furnival, and our readers Ms Fiona Plowman and Mrs Sarah Beanland. Our thanks also go to Mrs Deborah Gee who transcribed the seminar. Finally we thank the Wellcome Trust for supporting this programme.

Tilli Tansey

Lois Reynolds

Caroline Overy

School of History, Queen Mary, University of London

VOLUMES IN THIS SERIES

1. Technology transfer in Britain: The case of monoclonal antibodies
   Self and non-self: A history of autoimmunity
   Endogenous opiates
   The Committee on Safety of Drugs (1997)
   ISBN 1 86983 579 4

2. Making the human body transparent: The impact of NMR and MRI
   Research in general practice
   Drugs in psychiatric practice
   The MRC Common Cold Unit (1998)
   ISBN 1 86983 539 5

3. Early heart transplant surgery in the UK (1999)
   ISBN 1 84129 007 6

4. Haemophilia: Recent history of clinical management (1999)
   ISBN 1 84129 008 4

5. Looking at the unborn: Historical aspects of
   obstetric ultrasound (2000)
   ISBN 1 84129 011 4

6. Post penicillin antibiotics: From acceptance to resistance? (2000)
   ISBN 1 84129 012 2

7. Clinical research in Britain, 1950–1980 (2000)
   ISBN 1 84129 016 5

8. Intestinal absorption (2000)
   ISBN 1 84129 017 3

9. Neonatal intensive care (2001)
   ISBN 0 85484 076 1

43. **WHO Framework Convention on Tobacco Control (2012)**
ISBN 978 0 90223 877 0

44. **History of the Avon Longitudinal Study of Parents and Children (ALSPAC), *c*.1980–2000 (2012)**
ISBN 978 0 90223 878 7 (this volume)

All volumes are freely available online at www.history.qmul.ac.uk/research/modbiomed/wellcome_witnesses

Hard copies of volumes 21–44 can be ordered from www.amazon.co.uk; www.amazon.com; and all good booksellers for £6/$10 each plus postage, using the ISBN.

UNPUBLISHED WITNESS SEMINARS

1994   **The early history of renal transplantation**

1994   **Pneumoconiosis of coal workers**
(partially published in volume 13, *Population-based research in south Wales*)

1995   **Oral contraceptives**

2003   **Beyond the asylum: Anti-psychiatry and care in the community**

2003   **Thrombolysis**
(partially published in volume 27, *Cholesterol, atherosclerosis and coronary disease in the UK, 1950–2000*)

2007   **DNA fingerprinting**

The transcripts and records of all Witness Seminars are held in archives and manuscripts, Wellcome Library, London, at GC/253.

OTHER PUBLICATIONS

Technology transfer in Britain: The case of monoclonal antibodies
Tansey E M, Catterall P P. (1993) *Contemporary Record* **9**: 409–44.

Monoclonal antibodies: A witness seminar on contemporary medical history
Tansey E M, Catterall P P. (1994) *Medical History* **38**: 322–7.

Chronic pulmonary disease in South Wales coalmines: An eye-witness account of the MRC surveys (1937–42)
P D'Arcy Hart, edited and annotated by E M Tansey. (1998)
Social History of Medicine **11**: 459–68.

Ashes to Ashes – The history of smoking and health
Lock S P, Reynolds L A, Tansey E M. (eds) (1998) Amsterdam: Rodopi BV, 228pp. ISBN 90420 0396 0 (Hfl 125) (hardback). Reprinted 2003.

Witnessing medical history. An interview with Dr Rosemary Biggs
Professor Christine Lee and Dr Charles Rizza (interviewers). (1998)
Haemophilia **4**: 769–77.

Witnessing the Witnesses: Pitfalls and potentials of the Witness Seminar in twentieth century medicine
Tansey E M, in Doel R, Søderqvist T. (eds) (2006) *Writing Recent Science: The historiography of contemporary science, technology and medicine.* London: Routledge: 260–78.

The Witness Seminar technique in modern medical history
Tansey E M, in Cook H J, Bhattacharya S, Hardy A. (eds) (2008) *History of the Social Determinants of Health: Global Histories, Contemporary Debates.* London: Orient Longman: 279–95.

Today's medicine, tomorrow's medical history
Tansey E M, in Natvig J B, Swärd E T, Hem E. (eds) (2009) *Historier om helse* (*Histories about Health,* in Norwegian). Oslo: *Journal of the Norwegian Medical Association:* 166–73.

INTRODUCTION

Those of us concerned with medical and biological research (and its funding) need to consider many factors: a long memory, a conscience, willingness to work round mindless rules and regulations, and a disdain for action that is not backed by evidence. Some are occasionally ignored. The Avon Longitudinal Study of Pregnancy and Childhood (now known as The Avon Longitudinal Study of Parents and Children) – ALSPAC – illustrates these points to a nicety.

The lament for the days when research was one man (usually a man) and his ideas, alone in his clinic or laboratory, is almost silent. It is even less likely, one might argue, that a major epidemiological study could be born from the ideas and drive of one person. ALSPAC is the counter-argument. Those with the aforementioned long memory, who can recall Jean Golding's determined advocacy of ALSPAC some 30 years ago, will agree that the impelling force of one well-prepared and well-informed individual was essential for the inception, growth and long life of the project. That drive and determination is well recognised by the participants at this seminar.

Should this account trouble our consciences? One reason why it might is eloquently described by participants in the seminar. Once the scientific merit of ALSPAC had been agreed after careful peer review, why was it so difficult for the essential infrastructure to be created? Why did funding agencies persist in the style of Procrustes, attempting to fit the funding of ALSPAC into the project grant model? Nevertheless, the fact is that funding was found. The Wellcome Trust, to its great credit, recognized the strength of the scientific case made by Jean Golding, and provided her personal support for many years, at a time when the Trust was much less wealthy than it is now. An increase in the resources of the Trust allowed more complete funding, including support for the infrastructure.

The moral that emerges for the funder is that if a piece of research deserves financial support, and if the funder has enough money, then a form of funding must be found – or created – to deliver that funding. Persuading other funding agencies to provide infrastructure or other core funding should, for the researcher, not be a distraction from the struggle to ensure that good work gets done. In the case of ALSPAC, only the vision of the leaders of the University of Bristol, and the strong nerves of its finance department, kept the project alive.[1]

---

[1] See comments by Professor Brian Pickering and Professor Gordon Stirrat on pages 18–19.

Even when it has been carefully designed, research often develops in unplanned ways. One of the plans for ALSPAC, from the start, was to collect biological samples, which was unusual in large cohort studies at that time. Meticulous attention to sample collection, documentation and storage, and the linkage to other survey data, questionnaires and so on, has created a treasure trove for research both now and in the future. But who could have predicted that genetic information, rather than biological or biochemical data, would be the main achievement to date? These achievements in genetics from ALSPAC epitomise the current weakness in matching biological understanding to the cornucopia of genetic information, a challenge for twenty-first century biological science.

To return to the opening list of precepts, there is the question of rules and regulations, some of which certainly appear mindless. Again, long memories will recall a time when patients and populations in research were protected mainly by the conscience and professional standards of the scientist or doctor conducting research and by the common law of tort. Are we really better off for the regulations that now surround us, on, for example, consent?[2] It certainly is not logical for large-scale clinical trials or cohort studies, with a single precise protocol, to be seen by multiple ethics committees, and sometimes to face different requirements in different places.[3] Research ethics is not a matter that should have geographical variation within one country. ALSPAC led rather than followed here: its Ethics Committee was set up very early in the project, and promoted the intelligent development of the legal and ethics framework of the study.[4] The regulations and procedures for gaining ethics approval for large-scale epidemiological research must be clear and consistent. Similarly, the rules for the use of National Health Service facilities for clinical and epidemiological research (for example, for support from the National Institute for Health Research Clinical Research Network[5]) must be clear and appropriate. As I have argued before, the NHS – "…a population-wide, comprehensive healthcare system, free to the patient at the point of consultation, and able to support the clinical infrastructure of research…"[6] is a research resource almost without rival, worldwide, and must remain open and accessible to good quality epidemiological and clinical studies.

---

[2] See comments by Professor Catherine Peckham on page 49.

[3] See comments by Professor George Davey Smith on pages 75–6.

[4] See comments by Mrs Elizabeth Mumford on pages 71–5.

[5] http://www.crncc.nihr.ac.uk/about_us/processes/portfolio (visited 16 April 2012).

[6] http://www.history.qmul.ac.uk/research/modbiomed/Publications/wit_vols/44829.pdf page i (visited 16 April 2012).

ALSPAC has implications for the funding, and for the regulatory framework of other major epidemiological studies. It sits alongside other pioneering population studies, such as the National Perinatal Mortality Surveys,[7] and shows that the field remains open for well-planned studies, often to answer specific hypotheses, but also with the potential to unlock important new and unexpected information. ALSPAC has created data that provides sound evidence for our understanding of child development. As the evidence supporting science and medicine grows, should not associated decisions be equally based on strong evidence? What, for example, is the economic, social and epidemiological evidence that supports successive reorganizations of health care systems? Are the changes introduced to medical education always based on reasonable evidence, rather than guesswork? Medicine, biomedical science, or medical education should never become like climate science, distorted by ideological argument: evidence matters.

ALSPAC has handsomely rewarded those who had the vision to create the project, and to provide the funding, and has given us solid new scientific information. This Witness Seminar tells its story, so far.

David Gordon
World Federation for Medical Education

[7] See http://cls.ioe.ac.uk/page.aspx?&sitesectionid=736&sitesectiontitle=Perinatal+Mortality+Survey+(1958 (visited 16 April, 2012).

HISTORY OF THE AVON LONGITUDINAL STUDY OF PARENTS AND CHILDREN (ALSPAC), c.1980–2000

The transcript of a Witness Seminar held by the History of Modern Biomedicine Research Group, Queen Mary, University of London, on 24 May 2011

Edited by C Overy, L A Reynolds and E M Tansey

HISTORY OF THE AVON LONGITUDINAL STUDY OF PARENTS AND CHILDREN (ALSPAC), c.1980–2000

Participants

Miss Karen Birmingham
Mrs Ruth Bowles
Dr Ian Lister Cheese
Professor George Davey Smith
Professor Alan Emond
Professor Jean Golding
Mrs Yasmin Iles-Caven
Dr Richard Jones
Mrs Elizabeth Mumford
Professor Catherine Peckham (chair)

Professor Marcus Pembrey
Professor Brian Pickering
Dr Jon Pollock
Dr Sue Ring
Mrs Sue Sadler
Professor Gordon Stirrat
Professor Tilli Tansey
Dr Linda Tyfield
Mr Mike Wall

Apologies include: Sir Iain Chalmers, Mr Ian Crawford, Dr Alan Doyle, Professor David Gordon, Dr Russell Hamilton, Professor Sir John Kingman, Professor Sir Alex Markham, Dr Charles Pennock, Ms Julie Wallis

Professor Tilli Tansey: Ladies and gentlemen, I'd like to begin by welcoming you all to this Witness Seminar on ALSPAC.[1] I'm the convenor of the History of Modern Biomedicine Research Group; and in the mid-1990s we started Witness Seminars to get together historians, scientists and clinicians who are interested in the history of medicine, as a way of getting to know each other but also to generate material resources in modern medical science and modern medical practice. We conduct a variety of meetings and you will see flyers of our meetings with the list of everything we've ever done. We transcribe and edit the proceedings of all our meetings. Everything is freely available on the web, and is downloadable. Nothing will be published from this meeting without your express written permission.

The subject of ALSPAC, the Avon Longitudinal Study of Parents and Children, was first mentioned to me as a possible Witness Seminar by Marcus Pembrey and Jean Golding several years ago, and it has taken some while to try to work out how and when to do it. We're delighted that we are finally holding it and, of course, a key person in any of these meetings is the chairman. We're particularly pleased that Catherine Peckham has agreed to chair this meeting. She's professor of paediatric epidemiology at the Institute of Child Health, and she is best known for her work on infections in pregnancy, particularly rubella, cytomegalovirus and HIV, and their impact on the fetus and development of the child. She showed that congenital rubella damage caused by exposure to maternal infection in pregnancy could continue after birth.[2] She's worked a lot on national cohort studies and therefore she's an absolutely ideal person to chair our meeting on ALSPAC; and without further ado I'll hand over to Catherine.

Professor Catherine Peckham: This is the first time I've experienced one of these Witness Seminars and it is like going back down memory lane. I remember that I first met Jean Golding in the 1960s when I was working on the 1958 cohort,[3] and working on cohorts in those days was considered very non-medical. You had to have a foot in the medical environment to be doing real research, and the cohorts were regarded as rather descriptive social research with little

---

[1]   The Avon Longitudinal Study of Parents and Children (also known as Children of the 90s). Until 1999 ALSPAC referred to the Avon Longitudinal Study of Pregnancy and Childhood.

[2]   See note 4.

[3]   The 1958 Birth Cohort or the National Child Development Study (NCDS) was initially designed to examine perinatal mortality among the children born in Great Britain in one week in March 1958. Although not designed as a longitudinal survey, a large proportion of the cohort has been followed since then. See Peckham (1973); Power and Elliott (2006) and Welshman (2012). See also Appendix 1.

Getting started:
Influences
Funding
Recruitment
early advisers
staff
participants

Themes and issues:
Collection of Biological Material
non genetic
genetic
Ethics

Table 1: Outline programme for 'History of the Avon Longitudinal Study of Parents and Children' Witness Seminar

relevance for medicine. However we all knew they were useful and important. My particular area of research was in infections in pregnancy, especially the adverse effects of infections in pregnancy on the child,[4] both in the near term and long term, and to me birth cohort studies were incredibly important. So it was a pleasure to have met people like Jean Golding. The analysis of data from these studies was then quite basic because we hadn't the technology that enabled us to do sophisticated analyses; a lot was done with counter sorters, and by hand, and it's been interesting looking at the evolution of these studies over time. That takes me to a discussion that I had at a meeting organized by Iain Chalmers in Oxford.[5] I'm sure you'll remember it, Jean. You talked to me about the need for a new cohort; the need to move from the birth of the child to understand more about what was going on in pregnancy. I thought this was a great idea because I had always been interested in events in pregnancy, and I was concerned we were relying on memory or recorded events or interventions in pregnancy, and not acquiring the necessary detailed information. It was an era when trials were everything: people wanted to do things scientifically, and cohort studies were not then regarded as scientific. We had an interesting discussion and I encouraged Jean to 'go for it!' I thought it was important and she had the necessary passion and energy. I think it's extraordinary that one person was able to fight against the system and be so far advanced in thinking about the issues.

---

[4] See, for example, Peckham (1972); Peckham *et al.* (1983, 1988).

[5] Sir Iain Chalmers directed the National Perinatal Epidemiology Unit in Oxford between 1978 and 1992.

I would like you to try to recall that meeting in Oxford, Jean, and to ask you to rehearse what you think the objectives were and why you thought this new study would progress the whole cohort development; how you justified it being local, not national, because people would say you can't extrapolate the findings to the general population. I'd like you to start there, telling us what your thoughts were; what was going on within the medical fraternity at the time – genetics wasn't the key issue – we were in an era when people were beginning to talk about the importance of early life on later health; people were talking a great deal about immunology. Can you tell us about the beginning and your ideas at that time?

Professor Jean Golding: Well, certainly the beginning for me was when I fortuitously started working with big, national cohort studies. So I'd worked on the 1958 cohort study[6] and fell in love with the methodology, and in particular, looking at things like congenital malformations, which I thought were fascinating, although not many other people did. And then when there was an opportunity, I was invited by Iain Chalmers to design a new national cohort study, and so I did a lot of thinking, talking to experts in various fields and came up with a design that involved enrolling mothers in pregnancy. Well, if you're doing a study nationally, enrolling in pregnancy and having a defined cohort is pretty difficult. But we decided it was do-able by enrolling a lot more people than you'd actually end up studying. So you'd get information on pregnancies in huge numbers. I've just been reading the document I produced, which I haven't read since 1980 and I was going for 50 000 deliveries to be followed up, plus some samples of different sorts, which perhaps rightly, was turned down out of hand.[7] But it had meant that I'd thought through the importance of pregnancy and thought through the importance of following up in detail, particularly looking at environmental factors in pregnancy, which had been very much ignored, other than smoking.[8] As things developed it was the importance of including biological samples that came to the fore as one of the ways of measuring environments that you couldn't measure in other ways. The next phase in all this, by which time I was in Bristol,[9] I was invited by WHO to a meeting in Moscow in 1985, which

---

[6] See note 3.

[7] Professor Jean Golding wrote: 'This was turned down by the Department of Health who had commissioned me to design and cost the study.' E-mail to Ms Caroline Overy, 18 December 2011.

[8] For the adverse effects of smoking in pregnancy see, for example, Simpson (1957); McIntosh (1984); Kleinman *et al.* (1988).

[9] Professor Jean Golding went to Bristol in 1980.

had a very vague remit but it was basically to design a study.[10] Because I was the only native English-speaker, I was the rapporteur. After talking round in circles for two or three days, I decided I would write what I thought they ought to have decided, rather than what they didn't decide, and presented that the next day. They all were enthusiastic, and so we developed it from there. I was slightly devious there, but [laughs] open in the end.

What we ended up with was the design of a cohort study which started in pregnancy and followed children through, long term. And because there was a very loquacious Greek psychologist there, there was a big emphasis on the psychology and the importance of measuring the psychology of the parents, and the way they interacted and the way they would interact with the child, and the child's behaviour.[11] So that helped formulate the design a lot. WHO, and this was only WHO EURO, so it was only the European countries,[12] decided that this warranted some piloting, so it gave me US $5000 to pilot, in Greece and Russia and the UK, to see whether one could collect accurate information using self-completed questionnaires. That was thought not to be the sort of thing that one did, you know, you wouldn't get accurate answers, you had to have trained interviewers. So we did pilot studies and compared results with things that we could validate to show what would work and what wouldn't work.[13] Well, we showed that it would be difficult to do it in Greece because we put the Eysenck psychology scale in there and that includes a lie scale, and they were scoring very high on the lie scale.[14] In other words, they were giving us the answers they thought we wanted. [Laughs] So that wasn't very good. The others, Russia and England,

---

[10] Professor Jean Golding wrote: 'WHO's remit was that the study should be undertaken across Europe with the aim of concentrating on the health of children.' E-mail to Ms Caroline Overy, 18 December 2011.

[11] Professor Jean Golding wrote: 'The psychologist was Thalia Dragonas, based in Athens at the Foundation for Research in Childhood. She is now a professor at the department of early childhood education at the University of Athens.' E-mail to Ms Caroline Overy, 18 December 2011. Dragonas' research focuses on psychological and social identities.

[12] In 1985 WHO EURO comprised: Albania, Austria, Belgium, Bulgaria, Czechoslovakia, Denmark, Finland, France, German Democratic Republic, Federal Republic of Germany, Greece, Hungary, Iceland, Ireland, Italy, Luxembourg, Malta, Monaco, Morocco, Netherlands, Norway, Poland, Portugal, Romania, San Marino, Spain, Sweden, Switzerland, Turkey, USSR, United Kingdom and Yugoslavia; see Grant (1985): i.

[13] Some of the pilot studies comparing Greece and the UK were published in Dragonas *et al.* (1992); Thorpe *et al.* (1992a and b).

[14] Professor Hans Jürgen Eysenck (1916–1997), a German-British psychologist who worked on intelligence and behaviour theory. For his psychology scale, see Eysenck and Eysenck (1975).

were fine on that. The Russians, however, didn't like the questions that had more than a yes/no answer; they really didn't like gradations of grey, whereas the Brits did want that. There were various technicalities that one had to sort out in order to get something that could be used in different countries. But WHO at that point decided that we could progress and they wrote to every health department in Europe saying there was this study, and they would encourage them to take part, what the rules of the study were, that there would be a core of information to be collected, and then each country could add whatever they wanted to that core.[15] The countries that had a private health service really found it very difficult to even think about this, and largely didn't take part.[16] The countries that said 'yes' were mainly in the old Eastern bloc, who just put it in their five-year plan; funding wasn't an issue; they had people employed, they had to keep doing something. That was fine but our timing was all wrong, perestroika[17] happened very rapidly, and people unexpectedly had to raise their own funds for the research. But some countries are still carrying on with that study.[18] What none of them wanted to do was collect biological samples,[19] which we decided was very important, and so the Avon side of ELSPAC,[20] which is known as ALSPAC, expanded the basic data to be collected to include biological samples, not so much because of genetics, although by the time we started I'd met Marcus Pembrey, but so that we could look at things that you couldn't get from questionnaires, so that included features of the environment, and things like infections and immunology. So that's the way it began. There were lots of different aspects to this. One of the things WHO had said in this letter that went to all the Ministries of Health, was that WHO wouldn't contribute any funding except something towards a meeting of directors

---

[15] The study was called ELSPAC – the European Longitudinal Study of Pregnancy and Childhood. It comprised over 40 000 children and their families followed in Great Britain, Isle of Man, the Czech Republic, Slovakia, Russia, Ukraine, and initially in Greece and Spain. See Golding (1989a).

[16] Professor Jean Golding wrote: 'This is why Greece had to drop out and countries such as Belgium and France declined to join.' E-mail to Ms Caroline Overy, 18 December 2011.

[17] Perestroika was the policy of political, economic and social restructuring in the Soviet Union, instituted by Mikhail Gorbachev in the mid-1980s.

[18] Ukraine, Czech Republic, Slovakia and Great Britain (as ALSPAC) and the Isle of Man.

[19] Professor Jean Golding wrote: 'This was partly for ethical reasons, but also a question of resources required to both collect and process and store such samples.' E-mail to Ms Caroline Overy, 18 December 2011.

[20] Professor Jean Golding wrote: 'There was an Avon side because I was based in Bristol which is the centre of what was the Avon area.' E-mail to Ms Caroline Overy, 18 December 2011.

of the study annually, which fizzled out quite soon.[21] The people who wanted to take part did get more and more enthusiastic about the whole thing, and I think a lot of chance events helped take it forward.

I'm sure Marcus will tell you how we met, which was totally unplanned. I was fortunate in that, in Bristol, two of my old colleagues from Oxford were appointed, so Gordon Stirrat came very soon after I did, and David Baum was then appointed as professor of child health, and Neville Butler retired.[22] The input from those three was extremely important at various times. Other contributions from around the country were important in making sure that we'd honed our ideas, because we were challenged at all points, I think, not only in the overall design of doing everything. My argument is: 'You can't look at one thing without taking account of all these other things, and how are you going to find out anything new anyway unless you study it?' This is what clinicians do: noticing who comes into their consulting rooms; they realize they've all got blue eyes or whatever, so... discoveries are not always made with a prior hypothesis. That didn't go down terribly well. [Laughs] But, now, in the days in which a genome-wide association study (GWAS)[23] works and genetic analyses are done, which are totally hypothesis-free, I think it has been recognized more and more that this is a viable way of doing things. So that's the way in which we planned it.

Peckham: Would anyone like to come in on that? Gordon, would you? You were involved very much in the early days in Bristol.

Professor Gordon Stirrat: Yes, I was involved from the very beginning. I had been a clinical reader in obstetrics and gynaecology in the University of Oxford when Jean was there, and was involved in her work. I was very interested in the work she was doing in, for example, record linkage studies etc. When I moved to Bristol, my research area was fetal development and feto-maternal

---

[21] Professor Jean Golding wrote: 'These meetings fizzled out at the point at which our main supporter in WHO EURO, Dr Prokorskas, changed position and his successors were not interested or committed to the study.' E-mail to Ms Caroline Overy, 18 December 2011.

[22] Professor Gordon Stirrat was appointed professor and head of department of obstetrics & gynaecology in the University of Bristol in 1982; Professor Neville Butler (1920–2007) was professor of child health, University of Bristol, from 1965 until 1985, and was succeeded by Professor David Baum (1940–99) who had been clinical reader in paediatrics at the University of Oxford.

[23] Genome-wide association studies (GWAS) are used to identify common genetic factors that influence health and disease. See, for example, Hardy and Singleton (2009) and also the factsheet on the website of the National Human Genome Research Institute at www.genome.gov/20019523 (visited 14 November 2011).

relations,[24] and it seemed to me that a study of pregnancy, which I thought was an extremely important part of the ultimate development of the child, was being neglected, because people measured the first day of life as being birth. I knew very well there was actually an awful lot that went on *in utero*, including environmental aspects and as a result of infection. This was music to my ears and I was really very strongly supportive.

There was a very interesting episode that occurred, and Jean didn't know about this until yesterday. Given that WHO were not going to be providing funds, and of course the imperative was to get funds, Neville Butler approached the Wellcome Trust and Medical Research Council (MRC). He was told by the Wellcome Trust that, yes, the idea was good but, since he was going to be retiring within a relatively short time (he retired in 1985, so this must have been some time in 1983/4), they didn't feel they could support the project unless it was backed by another department in the University of Bristol, where the head of that department was not going to be retiring as soon as Neville was. So he approached me about that and I came with him to the Wellcome Trust and we had a discussion with them. The funding was given on the basis of it being jointly held by the two departments, and I feel very proud that I was able to facilitate this funding. Interestingly enough, Neville managed to keep that rather quiet, but we won't say any more about that. However, these arrangements led to real problems with David Baum, Neville's successor, because he had not been given this information. It was great to have David Baum in Bristol and the situation was sorted out and wasn't a lasting problem.[25] From my point of view, I was very privileged to be a facilitator of the project, and feel that perhaps there was something I contributed that was crucial; but then, of course, the whole collection of data right from the beginning of pregnancy was right up my street. However, it was not without its problems by any means. One of the things I was really excited about, and perhaps will talk about that later, was the collection of placentas,[26] because we tend to throw placentas out; we think they're just 'baggage', whereas other cultures have very different ideas

---

[24] See, for example, Sunderland *et al.* (1981); Sargent *et al.* (1982).

[25] Professor Gordon Stirrat wrote: 'In subsequent discussion it became clear that this episode related to a bid for a Wellcome Senior Lectureship for Jean and not the ALSPAC project per se'. Note on draft transcript, 6 September 2011. Professor Jean Golding also wrote of this episode: 'Much of it is true but is related to a different piece of research, not ALSPAC.' Note on draft transcript, 3 October 2011.

[26] The terms 'placentas' and 'placentae' were both used during the Witness Seminar. For consistency in this transcript, we have used the term 'placentas'.

about what the placenta is.[27] For example, the Greeks called the placenta and the membranes deutera while the Romans called them the secundinae, both of which mean the 'second born'. There's still a huge amount of information in a warehouse somewhere incarcerated within the placentas which are still kept, which I think could add to the study even now.[28]

Peckham: What was the funding from the Wellcome for? Was that for Jean's fellowship or salary? It wasn't for the study, was it?

Golding: No, it wasn't for the study.[29] It was for a research assistant or research fellow working with me, who was Jon Pollock, and a secretary. As it was, they demanded that the university took over my funding; I'm sure it was Brian Pickering who had to negotiate with the Wellcome Trust at the time.

Peckham: So that was a pretty pivotal moment?

Golding: Yes.

Peckham: Does anyone else want to say anything else about those early days? You were going to say something, George, about a note. Do you want to read it out? I think it's interesting. I don't know how it relates to the timing, but I imagine it was quite early on.

Professor George Davey Smith: Yes, this was earlier than Jean and I remembered, so it took me a while to find this. It was in the News and Notes section of the *Lancet*, 26 August 1989,[30] in the days when people used to read journals. I obviously had nothing better to do than to read the News and Notes in the *Lancet*. It said:

> Study on factors influencing child health
>
> A Longitudinal Study of Pregnancy and Childhood (ALSPAC) is being planned by the University of Bristol and is due to start in 11 months' time. The aim is to determine which biological, environmental, social, genetic, psychological, and psychosocial factors are associated with the

---

[27] See, for example, Birdsong (1998).

[28] Professor Jean Golding wrote: 'As so often in this study, data and samples were collected and little interest was taken in them for many years. In the case of the placentas, it was not until 2010 – then two different research groups obtained funding to look at the placentas in some detail.' E-mail to Ms Caroline Overy, 24 February 2012.

[29] See note 25.

[30] Anon. (1989).

survival and health of the fetus, infant and child. The cohort will consist of all births in the three Avon health districts over a 12-month period, and women and their partners will be recruited to the study as soon as possible after confirmation of pregnancy. Collaboration with other research groups or individuals is being sought. Potential collaborators should contact Dr Jean Golding, Division of Epidemiology, Institute of Child Health … Bristol.'

Peckham: And what date was that?

Davey Smith: 26 August 1989.

Peckham: 1989. Had you funding by then? [Laughter]

Professor Marcus Pembrey: Because we've got to 1989 I thought I'd better chip in as to when I first met Jean. In January 1988 there was a meeting on child development in Athens, and I was asked to talk about genetic prediction and so on, and Jean was talking on some other subject there.[31] We met and she said 'Oh, I've got this study that I'm quite interested in' and within two weeks, I see from my old work diaries that have been kept, Jean had come to visit me on 5 February. I remember that meeting very well. She asked if I would be interested and prepared to help, and I know that there is a letter that I then sent saying: 'I'm very happy to help where I can but I can't commit very much time, but I'll do what I can.' And, of course, within about two months it was taking up about 50 per cent of my academic work. But I'll come back to the genetics of it at a later stage.[32]

Professor Alan Emond: In 1985 I was appointed as lecturer. I arrived at the same time as David Baum, and I distinctly remember in the beginning of 1986, Jean summoning me to her office. I was very much the young lecturer; I had just finished my doctorate and I was looking for my first post-doc study. Jean called me in and I felt a bit nervous because I wasn't sure what it was about. [Laughter] She said: 'Oh, I've got this new project, this new cohort study that I'm going to launch. I've just come back.' She told me about the meeting in Moscow, and said: 'I want a keen paediatrician to help run it.' I thought that I fitted that category, and offered to be the paediatric link for the burgeoning design of the study. This was actually very timely for me, because I was launching a

---

[31] NATO Advanced Research Workshop on Early Influences Shaping the Individual, 20–24 January 1988, Athens, Greece. The proceedings of this meeting were published in Doxiadis (ed.) (1989). Papers include Pembrey (1989) and Golding (1989b).

[32] See page 57 onwards.

small follow-up study of preterm infants, the Avon Preterm Follow-up Study.[33] In that study we looked at a cohort of preterm babies in the community so we were able to pilot a lot of the questionnaires, which were used in pregnancy in ALSPAC. Through Jean's help, we received a small amount of funding from the Department of the Environment, who were particularly interested in the environmental effects on babies' health. We used the same methodology, self-completion questionnaires, to capture environmental information and then we linked that to health outcomes in these babies. A lot of the environmental aspects in the ALSPAC questionnaires were piloted as part of that study. I can honestly say I was the first paediatrician to be involved and I went around proselytizing the value of longitudinal studies, because previously, for my doctorate, I worked with the MRC Sickle Cell Unit in Jamaica with Graham Serjeant and had been completely convinced about the value of longitudinal studies.[34] So I brought that experience and that enthusiasm with me to the beginning of ALSPAC.

Peckham: The drawing together of interested individuals has obviously been very important. Before you even got the funding and were launching the project, it became a reality. It's interesting that the emphasis on the external environment was a key justification for taking the samples. This was so different from the earlier cohorts in that an attempt was being made to measure environmental exposure. This made it novel. How did you, Jean, justify restricting the study to a local level, countering the argument that it should be national? Was that a problem?

Golding: I didn't think it was a problem. I think it's only a problem if you consider the survey as something that is going to give you the prevalence within a country. But the value of longitudinal surveys is in the longitudinal nature of them, so it shouldn't matter so much that this is only taking place in one area; it might not have environments that you are interested in, but it does have a lot of environments you can look at longitudinally to see what the effects are. I think that is an advantage rather than a disadvantage, because you can actually get a handle on what those environments are. You can go out and sample, whereas that would be much more difficult to do nationally. That's the sort of thing we did with a number of different environments that we were measuring like the

---

[33] The Avon Preterm Follow-up Study investigated the interaction of environmental and medical factors on the health of preterm infants, less than 32 weeks' gestation, born in Avon between 1 October 1987 and 30 November 1988; see Emond *et al.* (1997).

[34] Emond (1987). Dr Graham Serjeant was then the director of the MRC Laboratories (Jamaica) which operated the Sickle Cell Unit at the University of the West Indies, Kingston, Jamaica; he retired in 1999.

electric magnetic radiation, or air pollutants.[35] That's one argument for having it local, but the major advantage, I think, is that locally you can get your local media and all the local health professionals to become part of the study, to be interested in it and want to know what the latest results are. Nearly everybody who's lived in Bristol or the surrounding area knows somebody who's in the study. It's very unusual for me to meet somebody who doesn't tell me about their cousin or their nephew or a friend who is part of the study. I think that sort of drawing together of the community couldn't happen with a national study. They don't know one another, whereas here you have whole classes at school where nearly everybody in the class is part of the study, and those who aren't feel very jealous of those who are, which keeps the whole thing rolling along. So, there are major advantages to having it in one area.[36]

Peckham: It is very helpful to hear the case for the local study and local ownership. This has important implications for governance, which we'll talk about later.

Golding: One other thing about being local is the examination of children. You can do it under situations that you have control of. For example, if you're doing something simple like taking the blood pressure of children around the country, such as happened in the 1970 cohort, we had geographic differences between areas but didn't know if they were real geographic differences or differences between the people measuring the blood pressure.[37] We never sorted that one out, whereas in this case we can keep hands on and keep that aspect under control.

Peckham: Does anyone want to add anything at this point?

Dr Jon Pollock: I want to emphasize two scientific components of the origins of this study, which were very impressive for me in relation to the British birth cohort studies that had gone before, which many of us had worked on.[38] And that was Jean explaining to me, and me being convinced by, the argument that

---

[35] Preece *et al.* (1999); Sherriff *et al.* (2005).

[36] For a discussion of the use of a local rather than national sample, see Golding (2009).

[37] The 1970 British Cohort Study (BCS70) is an ongoing longitudinal study, which started by collecting data about the births and families of just under 17 200 babies born in the UK in one particular week in April 1970; see http://cls.ioe.ac.uk/page.aspx?&sitesectionid=795&sitesectiontitle=Welcome+to+the+1970+British+Cohort+Study (visited 31 January 2012). See also Elliott and Shepherd (2006).

[38] See notes 3 and 37.

longitudinal studies should be planned as longitudinal studies and the idea of funding a study to be longitudinal. Of course, the earlier national cohort studies were not longitudinal; they were cross-sectional studies that became longitudinal.[39] That's a much easier arrangement to have managerially, but, of course, it means that you're not necessarily collecting the right information at the right time, particularly in relation to measuring exposures close to the time of exposure, as opposed to retrospective recall of data, which is what largely they depend on.[40] That's one issue which, I think, makes this study unique, or rare, in the scientific literature. The other is an issue that you skated over, Jean, but I think we're going to have to come back to it, is the business of this not being a hypothesis-generated study. This was seen at the time to be a serious weakness of the study, particularly in relation to funding opportunities, of course. There are lots of good reasons for that, but, as time will tell, as things will happen, as the information emerges, there is a case to be argued for whether that was actually a weakness or a strength of the study. I think that that is a topic we could come back to. We didn't have any specific hypotheses. There may have been lots of individual hypotheses that would have been seen as answerable by the study, but there were no specific driving hypotheses in terms of child development, which became a key issue on which a funding bid could be put forward at an early stage.

Peckham: That is a comment that would apply even to the newly funded cohort.[41] I don't think you can say that it was without hypothesis, because Jean has already said it was based on the belief that intra-uterine life and environment had an important impact on outcome. In a sense that is a hypothesis. As there is not a single question, you have to keep the study quite broad. I would

---

[39] See Appendix 1.

[40] Dr Pollock wrote: 'The previous national birth cohort studies were planned to be single sweep cross-sectional studies. It might have been that researchers foresaw the opportunity for further longitudinal studies but they were not planned as such. When funding was later obtained for follow-ups, conducted usually several years later and which turned them into longitudinal studies, the sweeps probed past events some time retrospectively (as opposed to collecting information shortly after the events occurred as in ALSPAC). So, for example, data on infant feeding in the weeks and months after birth in the British Births Cohort 1970 study were not collected from the mother until the index child was 5 years old. The degree to which data are retrospectively collected is minimized, and hence data quality higher, when longitudinal studies are planned to be so.' E-mail to Ms Caroline Overy, 7 December 2011.

[41] The 2012 Birth Cohort Study, funded by the Department of Business Innovation and Skills (BIS), the Economic and Social Research Council (ESRC) and the Medical Research Council (MRC), will be the largest UK-wide study of babies and young children, and will follow 90 000 children and their families from pregnancy through to the early years; see www.esrc.ac.uk/funding-and-guidance/tools-and-resources/research-resources/surveys/bcf.aspx (visited 30 November 2011).

have thought that this applied to all the birth cohorts, and I know it's often a controversial issue. Going back to the discussion about funding, although in the minds of those who created the 1958 birth cohort study, and other similar studies, the overall concept was longitudinal and long term, nobody is likely to give you money for something that is very protracted. Even for the most recent new cohort currently being planned, funding is only for the first two years. Of course, the expectation is that it will go on for much longer. I think it's very hard to build long-term funding into these studies. I remember discussions about the 1958 cohort when we were trying to raise funds for the follow-ups. In meetings in the Department of Health we had to look at each question to determine whether it was relevant to the longitudinal nature of the study rather than information which could have been gathered in a 'single sweep'. There was a great deal of discussion to ensure that the cross-sectional data not essential to the study was excluded. I think that such discussions are extremely important to keep the studies tight. This brings us onto the funding. Jean, you've gone a long way without any funding. Can you tell me, what next?

Golding: We got $5000 for piloting.[42] [Laughter]

Peckham: But at least you'd got your salary to be able to bring everyone on board.[43] How did you get the first funding for the study?

Golding: Well, the ideal which we tried to work towards was to get a consortium of funders to all put in a certain amount of funding to get the thing going.

Peckham: What sort of funders?

Golding: Government departments, research councils, particularly the MRC, and charities, Asthma UK, or whatever it was called then;[44] Action Research;[45] a huge number of different charities that were interested. The first thing we did to

---

[42] See page 6.

[43] See page 10 and note 25

[44] Asthma Research Council (ARC) was founded in 1927 to conduct research into the 'cause and cure of asthma from a firm scientific foundation.' In 1989 this merged with the fundraising 'Friends of the ARC' to form the National Asthma Campaign; this became Asthma UK in 2004; www.asthma.org.uk/index.html (visited 31 January 2012).

[45] Action Research (Action Medical Research since 2003) was founded in 1952 as the National Fund for Poliomyelitis with the aim of finding a cure for polio. With the introduction of the vaccine and subsequent reduction in the disease, the charity changed its emphasis to include other crippling diseases. Today, its aim is to fund medical research 'to help stop the suffering of babies and children caused by disease and disability'; www.action.org.uk/ (visited 31 January 2012).

start with, I should say the most important thing we did, was to form a steering committee, which had important people like you [Catherine Peckham] on it, and Marcus Pembrey, Gordon Stirrat and David Baum, and Michael Rutter.[46] We (i.e. the Steering Committee) worked towards having a meeting of all this group of potential funders and that was held in August 1989. The MRC hosted it and there was a good turnout of various government departments and two people from the MRC, and different charities. Some of the participants are here today: Ian Lister Cheese was there; Alan Emond was there; also Yasmin Iles-Caven, who was my PA at the time; Marcus Pembrey, Jon Pollock and Gordon Stirrat. We presented the idea of ALSPAC and what it could do for government departments and various people, hoping that we were going to end up with, you know, quantities of long-term funding. We ended up with a basic: 'well, it's a really positive idea', but my memory of what they said was that it couldn't be done in that way, it had to be done with project grants. Somehow the project grants would be focused on specific questions and we were expected to be able to juggle the money so it would pay for the long-term project.

Peckham: So then you had to develop your hypotheses? [Laughter]

Golding: And how… yes. And there were various people at that meeting, who did have their own hypotheses that they wanted us to look at. Those from the Department of the Environment were the strongest ones. They'd always wanted to be able to access homes so they could measure air pollutants indoors and they hadn't got a mechanism for doing so; and we could be the mechanism, which fitted in with our study of the environment and how we could do it. So, that was fine. We won grants here and there, but didn't have quite enough to feel comfortable about starting, when I got this phone call from the Department of the Environment saying: 'Why haven't you started yet? We've started employing the people who are going to do the measurements.' [Laughter] We were squeezed, so we had to start, because we'd got their money. I mean, maybe we could have said 'no', but anyway we were kick-started.

Peckham: So how did you start without any money?

Golding: Well, we had some money. We had enough to keep us going until December 1991, which I remember well. I think most of us remember it well, particularly the people who were employed because that's the point at which we

---

[46] Professor Sir Michael Rutter (b. 1933) is professor of developmental psychopathology at the Institute of Psychiatry, King's College, London. He set up the MRC Child Psychiatry Research Unit in 1984 and the Social, Genetic and Developmental Psychiatry Unit at the Institute of Psychiatry in 1994.

were definitely in the red as far as the university was concerned. And it was, you know, a big drop. The Steering Committee had seen it coming, and we'd been talking about it month after month, and writing grants galore, some of which we won, but it was never quite enough. That was the point at which the first furore happened at the Department of Child Health in Bristol, which Alan, I think, remembers well. Do you want to speak about that, because I wasn't quite aware of what was going on?

Emond: Most of the paediatricians knew that ALSPAC was being run on a wing and a prayer, and there was a bit of disquiet, but I think Jean had an aura about her that people believed that she would come through. And I think Jean's greatest characteristic is her dogged optimism that things will come right. That inspired people like me to follow, but some of her senior colleagues were less sanguine about it. A note came down from higher up in the university that ALSPAC was in the red, and shortly after that came an open threat from finance that they were going to freeze all the senior academics' discretionary funds to pay for the ALSPAC debt.[47] I'll never forget the reaction of my seniors – it was quite an eye-opener for me as a young academic about the way that the seniors behaved, because people just came out of the woodwork – I won't mention names, but some of my senior colleagues appeared out of nowhere, livid that the pot of discretionary money that they'd been building up over the years could just go to pay for Jean Golding's irresponsible debt. [Laughter] This was a major ruction that actually took some time to heal between the different academic paediatricians, and I'll never forget it. We were saved because of Sir John Kingman, the vice-chancellor at the time, who is a statistician and really understood the value of longitudinal studies.[48] I think Jean had lunch with him on a regular basis.

Golding: No, I didn't.

Emond: Well, that was my fantasy anyway! [Laughter] That you somehow got Sir John on side and that saved our bacon. But the project very nearly went down the tubes.

---

[47] See pages 22–3.

[48] Sir John Kingman was vice-chancellor of Bristol University from 1985 to 2001 and was president of the Royal Statistical Society from 1987 to 1989.

Golding: I think it was getting Brian onside particularly.

Peckham: The university role and support was clearly important. Certainly the steering group was very aware of that. Brian, would you like to say something about that?

Professor Brian Pickering: My memory is very, very hazy of those times. In 1992, I became the deputy vice-chancellor of the University of Bristol. One of my jobs was to have oversight of the allocation of the university resources. So in fact it was me that Jean naturally tried to persuade, and we had a number of conversations at the time. There was, of course, a great feeling in the university that while university funds should be used to provide, as it was called then, the Well-Found Laboratory, and then also to pump prime. If a project, in its broadest sense, was to be viable, then outside funds had to be found.[49] What we were doing at that time, from 1992 on, was actually trying to keep the wolf not just from the door, but from actually beginning to bite in the sitting room! As Alan said, clearly there was support from my boss, the vice-chancellor, who appreciated the importance of longitudinal studies; and in many respects, was in favour of long-term funding rather than of individual project grants.

While there was general support for the ALSPAC activity by funders, there was a reluctance to fund the individual project grant applications. I think it came back to the 'hypothesis' situation and 'fishing expeditions', which were comments that were heard from time to time.

In the university, too, there was general support for ALSPAC, and we felt that we ought to try and make sure that it was able to survive until it got long-term funding from outside. Of course, university funds are finite: if one feeds Peter, there are lots of Pauls who have to give up some of the crumbs and their hidden criticism is present all the time. As the academic in charge, I was helped by the enormous support of the finance director, Ian Crawford, who is down as an 'apology' today.[50] Ian felt that ALSPAC activities could be considered as good

---

[49] At that time university research was funded by the 'dual support system', in which core support for general purposes was allocated by the University Grants Committee (replaced by the University Funding Council in 1989, and in 1992 by the Higher Education Funding Council for England) and project-specific funds were gained from grants awarded by research councils, charities and industry. A report by the Advisory Board for the research councils (ABRC) in 1987 states: 'University money for the support of research serves two purposes. On the one hand it provides for a basic level of research activity for all university academic staff. On the other hand it provides the "well-found" laboratory in which work supported by the Research Council and other funding agencies can be undertaken'. ABRC (1987), quoted in Adams and Bekhradnia (2004): 19.

[50] Mr Ian Crawford joined the University of Bristol in 1990 and retired as finance director in December 2008.

investments: Jean and her colleagues were likely to be developing techniques that the university could patent in time, and, in straight business terms, it was good to keep this project going. This was not something that was discussed openly in the university, but was his personal view, which of course, made my job a little easier when I wanted to say 'yes' to Jean, rather than 'no'. However, it became apparent that there was no pressure on anybody else outside to fund ALSPAC if the University of Bristol was doing it. I do remember coming to London with Jean, and indeed with Ian Crawford – the Wellcome Trust facilitated and hosted a meeting at which there were representatives of MRC, the Department of Health (DoH) and such like.[51] I remember taking a rather histrionic line that it was not for the University of Bristol to fund the future of the nation's health. There were other people there but, I think largely with support from the Wellcome Trust, a great deal of good came out of that meeting, and there was then a movement into calmer, if not really calm, waters.

It seems to me, listening to the discussion earlier on that, perhaps with hindsight, this was an adversity that had a sweet use, because if there had been national DoH funding from the beginning, then there would have been an enormous amount of pressure to actually widen the study nationally, which would have lost the compactness that Jean was talking about, from keeping it in Avon.

Stirrat: If I may just add something. Of course, for this study to succeed there had to be a considerable infrastructure, it could not have functioned otherwise. Unfortunately the project grant model, which was dogmatically pursued by the funders, actually caused us huge headaches, because there was an absolute refusal to even consider the possibility that they should actually contribute to the infrastructure – this wasn't the same as co-funding. This persisted for many years and came very close to scuppering the whole thing on several occasions. It really was only by dint of the university's generosity and the foresight of, for example, Brian Pickering and Ian Crawford, that it was overcome. I think there's a lesson to be learned there.

Peckham: I think that's important because at the time there was quite a lot of criticism that you were driven to do the studies that got the funding, rather than the studies that needed to be done. That was a major criticism that came from outside.

---

[51] Mrs Yasmin Iles-Caven wrote: 'The date of the meeting was 29 March 1999.' E-mail to Ms Caroline Overy, 13 February 2012.

Pembrey: I want to contribute a little bit to the funding situation at that time, because we'll come back to the reason why we had decided that we ought to have transformed cell lines made from either the cord blood or subsequent blood samples. On 21 August 1989, one month before that meeting, the MRC meeting that we've heard about where everybody was there,[52] I went to see Joe Smith, the head of the Public Health Laboratory Service in Colindale.[53] It was a sunny day like today. I remember 9 o'clock in the morning I arrived there. Three-quarters of an hour later, I came out having been promised £200 000 of cell line activity under the guidance of Alan Doyle, who sadly could not be present today, who was then running the cell line facility at Porton Down.[54] I came out and thought: 'Well, that's a breeze! £200K, three-quarters of an hour', you know. [Laughter] My optimism really shot right up to the top, and I thought: 'Now it's going to be easy to get stuff from the MRC and the Wellcome Trust, because if we've got all this on board…' [Laughter] Not at all. That was

---

[52] See page 16.

[53] The Public Health Laboratory Service (PHLS) is now part of the Health Protection Agency (HPA); the HPA Colindale services include specialist and reference microbiology services and infectious disease surveillance; see www.hpa.org.uk/AboutTheHPA/WhoWeAre/CentreForInfections (visited 15 December 2011). Sir Joseph Smith became director of the Public Health Laboratory Service in August 1985, having previously been senior lecturer in bacteriology and immunology at the London School of Hygiene and Tropical Medicine. He retired in 1992.

[54] Dr Alan Doyle went on to become science programme manager at the Wellcome Trust with responsibility for a range of major research projects, such as longitudinal cohort studies including UK Biobank and the UK birth cohort studies. He is currently director of the National Information Governance Board for Health and Social Care. Dr Doyle wrote: 'The European Cell Bank at Porton Down had been established with initial Department of Trade and Industry funding in 1984 and the Epstein-Barr virus (EBV) transformed cell line facility commenced as a result of specific EC funding in 1986 based upon the technology I had gained experience of at the UK Transplant laboratories in Bristol in 1981–84. The overall remit of the Cell Bank was to provide services to the medical research community but this had to be done on a cost recovery basis. When approached by Professor Pembrey and Professor Golding, estimates of cost for generating cell lines from cord blood were discussed and submitted to the potential research funders and the subsidy from the parent organisation PHLS would have contributed significantly in reducing the overheads. Unfortunately at that particular period there was a significant and influential "anti-cell line lobby" amongst the scientific community who viewed this as an unnecessary extravagance and far too expensive to justify almost regardless of context. It was a decade or more later that whole genome association studies became dependent on large quantities of DNA only available from cell lines derived from donor lymphocytes. The Cell Bank at Porton continues on with this type of support work to this day. Having said that of course creating this resource at the outset would have been much more efficient and cost effective. It was somewhat ironic to me that the investment required to create the cell line resource from ALSPAC participants was approved by a scientific review conducted by the Wellcome Trust and MRC in 1999/2000 after I joined WT as a programme manager.' E-mail to Ms Caroline Overy, 13 February 2012.

a little blip, thinking that it was going to be straightforward. Then it was back into the grind. We didn't really get any funding on DNA until 1995, and for cell lines until 2001.

Peckham: So, Jean, when did it become viable? Did the funding problem, at least, enable you to know that you could carry on for a year without being in the red?

Golding: It certainly wasn't viable when we carried on. I think I was producing business plans on a monthly basis. We were producing lists of grants that were submitted, with my estimation of what the odds were of getting that particular money, which actually, if you multiplied the odds by the amount you'd applied for, and added it up, it came to what we got, but it might not have been the grants that we thought were going to be easy. This was the sort of system that we had in place, and you know, meetings every month, I think, certainly with the finance director. But the thing to be remembered is the effect on the staff, because we didn't have money: all our staff, or almost all the staff, were on contracts that lasted a month; they got their notice before they got their contract for the next month; and then, you know, you couldn't advertise for a post with that sort of funding anyway. We had so much loyalty and enthusiasm. It was: 'Well, we'll hear later…' It was just amazing.

Peckham: It was extraordinary. I don't think that would be possible now.

Golding: I think you can get the enthusiasm, and if you've got the staff already on board, I don't see why it's not possible. I hope you don't have to try it. One of the things that we did at that point when we went into the red, was to go to William Waldegrave, who happened to be the MP for our area, and he was the Minister of Health at the time, I think, or he had been the Minister of Health.[55] Anyway, he knew about ALSPAC, I'd seen him before and he raised questions with the Department of Health, who took it seriously, but decided not to core fund us. But, we were trying all sorts of things. One of the business plans that I developed was 'worse scenario, we stop now'; or put another way, 'extreme scenario number 1: we stop everything now'. The downside of that was that not only did you never pay the debt back, but you would also have to pay back that money given to you that you'd already spent on collecting data.

---

[55] William Waldegrave was Secretary of State for Health from 1990 until 1992, and MP for Bristol West from 1979 until 1997. He became Baron Waldegrave of North Hill in 1999.

That came to about minus £250 000 that you'd never pay back. The other extreme was to carry on working without having the full funding to do so, on the understanding that the money will come in. I prophesied that it would take five years to get in the black again.[56] I was wrong. [Laughter] But it got better, and you know, that's how we carried on, but it was really John Kingman, Brian Pickering and Ian Crawford, particularly, that kept it going. And I think one of the important things was a key part of a cohort study: if you stop collecting data as the babies were being born because you had run out of funds, and then caught up with them much later, you'd wasted that vital period of time, and the important information that should have been collected.

Mrs Yasmin Iles-Caven: I was Jean's PA for a very long time and then the resources manager for ALSPAC, so I know a lot about the figures and the trials and tribulations. I can clearly remember the day in early 1990 or so, when Jean called all the secretaries and me into a room and said: 'We're going to do this big study where we send out lots of questionnaires, write lots of grant applications, and we don't have a budget.' At the time, I think we were all really overwhelmed at the thought of all the extra work and that we didn't actually have the money to finance it, but little did we know. That was in the days before we had PCs, so we were hand-typing these grant applications. Going back to when they almost shut us down in 1991: we'd already had funding – about £2 million – invested in the development and the first 15 months of the project, and our predicted shortfall was about £53 000, which doesn't sound a lot of money now, but that was when things were really dire and they were going to close us down after Christmas.[57] I should say that our debt later rose to £1.5 million or so, which we managed to pay back over a number of years through the indirect income we'd won on grants being diverted to pay it off. But it was a huge risk for the university. For the finance director at the time, Ian Crawford, to take that kind of risk was amazing and showed how much he believed in the study. By about

---

[56] Professor Jean Golding wrote: 'It was never in the black, but once I had left, the university wrote off the debt.' E-mail to Ms Caroline Overy, 20 December 2011.

[57] Mrs Yasmin Iles-Caven wrote: 'We'd been told not to spend or commit any more monies as we were £53 000 over spent already. A large number of staff who worked as interviewers or 'Focus' clinic staff were hourly paid on a casual fee claims basis and their December claims would increase that overspend by at least £10 000. I believe our head of department and his departmental manager were considering asking the 'casual' staff not to come back after Christmas. This would have meant the closure of the Focus clinics and no one to mail out questionnaires or encourage participation. Disaster was averted thanks to Jean, who hand wrote a long letter to the vice-chancellor, which she personally delivered across the garden gate at his residence during the Christmas holidays.' E-mail to Ms Caroline Overy, 19 December 2011.

1993, we'd estimated the running costs were going to be about £1 million a year because we had 70 or more staff at the time, full- and part-time, and were sending our questionnaires to about 15 000 families. So it was a real hand-to-mouth existence. But we managed to beg, borrow – not quite steal – a lot of support in kind, like the university allowing us to use premises rent-free; the local hospitals allowed us to use space in their freezers to store biosamples and placentas; and we were able to get companies like Oral B to give toothbrushes as thank you gifts to the 'Children in Focus' groups.[58] Alongside ALSPAC, of course, we were trying to run ELSPAC at the same time. We tried obtaining funding from the EU on several occasions, which had pretty tight deadlines. I can remember travelling to Brussels by train and ferry to deliver applications on time. We got some money from the National Institutes of Health (NIH) to cover costs in places like Russia and the Ukraine. By about the early 1990s, one-third of our income came from government bodies and 20 per cent from charities, another 20 per cent from the commercial sector, and the rest from the USA (NIH and the March of Dimes).[59] But we did spend most of our time writing grant applications and fundraising letters, and we didn't do too badly, really, I think. I have got quite a lot of numbers, as I've been archiving all the old grants and failed submissions, and of those grants awarded between 1989 and 2005, approximately, we won 176 grants and more than 258 applications failed.[60]

Peckham: That's quite a high hit rate.

Iles-Caven: Yes, not bad.

Peckham: We ought to move on now to recruitment. It will be very interesting to know how you involved the local community; how you recruited the families. Who would like to talk about that?

---

[58] Ten 'Children in Focus' clinics were held at various time intervals between the ages of 4 and 61 months, using a 10 per cent sample of the cohort selected at random from the last six months of ALSPAC births. Further annual Focus Clinics were held from ages 7–17 years which were open to all study children. For a list of funding contributions towards the 'Children in Focus' study by 1997, see Appendix 3.

[59] The March of Dimes Foundation was set up in 1938 in the United States by President F D Roosevelt as the National Foundation for Infantile Paralysis (NFIP) to combat polio. In 1958, following the introduction of the Salk vaccine and the decline of the disease, the Foundation's mission changed to focus on the prevention of birth defects, infant mortality and premature birth, and now has the broader goal of improving the health of all pregnant women and babies; see www.marchofdimes.com/ (visited 25 January 2012).

[60] See Appendix 4 for revised figures.

Golding: I shall start by saying that one of our most important sources of recruitment was people knocking on the door to be members of staff. Sue Sadler, who is here, did that; and that was very valuable, because they already wanted to take part.

Peckham: How did they know about it?

Mrs Sue Sadler: I became the manager of the clinics after a couple of years of being with ALSPAC. I'd been a teacher and an antenatal teacher for some years and, between jobs and at a low ebb, a friend said: 'Do you know about this study that Jean Golding's doing?' And she talked about it. 'Why don't you contact her?' I thought: 'What a brilliant idea.' It sounded absolutely fabulous. So I did, and said, basically, not quite 'give us a job',[61] you know, but 'could I possibly come and help?' Jean wrote back saying, 'Well, tell me what you can do and some things you've written', and I did and lo and behold, I got a job. I think it doesn't happen anymore like that. There I was doing all sorts of jobs that were required before we eventually started running the clinics.

If you want to know a bit more about recruitment from my perspective, I then had to take on people to examine the babies, the newborns, first of all to measure the newborns and later during the actual clinic. You can't advertise even if you have the money, to give people jobs measuring newborns in hospital. It's a very special thing to do. I was in a fortunate position because I'd been working with the National Childbirth Trust[62] for a long time, and I knew the network, and knew this extremely valuable post-natal support set-up they have, where people who have been through the classes will then get together – sort of coffee mornings, what have you – but it's a group of people whom I felt were the kind of people that I wanted to be talking to new mums, and handling these newborn babies. That's how we got our first staff. It was word of mouth. I approached the organizers and asked: 'Have you got people who want a job who will be suited to doing this kind of thing?' and they came.[63] When we wanted

---

[61] 'Gizza job' (Give us [me] a job) was the catchphrase of the Liverpudlian character Yossa Hughes in the BBC television drama *Boys from the Blackstuff* (1982).

[62] Founded in 1956 as the National Childbirth Association, the National Childbirth Trust (NCT) obtained charitable status in 1961 and is now the largest UK parenting charity, offering antenatal and post-natal discussion classes, support groups and telephone support lines.

[63] Mrs Sue Sadler wrote: 'They did have to get through an interview first!' Note on draft transcript, 18 August 2011.

staff for the new Focus Clinics[64] from four months onwards, it was the same network of people and also people who were known by those already working for us. Nepotism, absolutely. But it worked because we had a very special kind of group of people who were very good with children and babies and mothers, and knew what it was like and could communicate well.

Peckham: How did you enrol the families? And involve the community?

Mrs Ruth Bowles: I'm a study mother. When I was asked to come along to this meeting I thought: 'I can't actually quite remember how I was enrolled!' So I asked around and, coming back to the point of it being a local study, I had plenty of people I could ask because they are my contemporaries – all our children were involved in the study. So that's another good reason for having it held locally, or in a distinct area. I was involved, and I was beginning to doubt my own memory, until Alan Emond spoke. In 1987 I remember taking part in a pilot study with my first child. I was handed a questionnaire in the hospital after he was born. I don't remember much more about it apart from answering the questions and putting comments on saying: 'Don't make me read all the questions unless I'm going to answer them. You know, put guides to say, "If you've answered no, move on to page 22" you know, because they were big booklets.' I think that must be Alan's fault, that one. [Laughs] In terms of being recruited with my study child, my third child, as I say I don't remember seeing any literature. My sister could remember quite clearly seeing literature up in the GP clinic and also the midwives mentioning it. She was attending a GP preconception clinic as a diabetic. But other friends also don't remember, but we eventually realized that we must have been asked beforehand, and when I looked through some papers of mine, I have actually got a letter here which says: 'Dear Mother-to-be…' so I guess I was asked before the baby was actually born (see Figure 1).

The other difficulty with that is that my third child was born at home, without the midwife or the GP. They came along a bit later on, so I don't know what actually happened to the placenta or anything like that; whether that was kept or taken away. But ALSPAC found me and I answered questions from then on. Other friends, as I say, remember being approached perhaps by a midwife at some point, and so I think the midwives were probably the key people, pre-birth, for enrolling most of the study mothers.

---

[64] See note 58.

The Avon Longitudinal Study of Pregnancy and Childhood
(ALSPAC)

Children of the Nineties
Institute of Child Health
University of Bristol
24 Tyndall Avenue
Bristol, BS2 8BJ

Tel: Hotline (0272) 256260
Tel: Office   (0272) 225967

Dear Mother-to-be,

    I am now enclosing the environment questionnaire from the Children of the Nineties study. As you will know, from the leaflet that we sent you recently, there is no obligation at all on you to fill this in. However, it would help us enormously if you were able to fill this in and send it back to us as soon as possible. One of the problems in trying to run a big survey of this sort is in ensuring that we don't send reminders to people who have already returned their questionnaires. Therefore the faster you return the questionnaire the better we will be able to cope with that problem.

    Remember, however, if you have any problems with the questionnaire - please let us know. You can contact us on the hotline or write me a note.

    With very best wishes and many thanks for your cooperation.

    Yours sincerely,

Jean Golding

Dr. Jean Golding
Director: Children of the Nineties.

Steering Committee:
Professor J. D. Baum, Professor G. M. Stirrat,
Professor M. Pembrey, Professor C. Peckham, Dr J. Golding,
Professor M. Rutter, Dr. C. Pennock, Dr. J. I. Pollock.

Figure 1: Letter sent to ALSPAC parents in 1990–92 during pregnancy and accompanying their first questionnaire.[65]

---

[65] The questionnaire referred to, 'Your Environment', may be downloaded at www.bristol.ac.uk/alspac/documents/ques-m01-your-environment.pdf (visited 17 January 2012).

Stirrat: Yes, I can confirm that, because it certainly was mainly the midwives, and in my position as the professor of obstetrics and gynaecology I was able to talk to our midwives in Bristol Maternity Hospital, as it was then, now St Michael's, and also in Southmead. We were able to make sure that there was a good lot of publicity for the study and a great willingness to be involved. There was an enthusiasm, it somehow or other just caught the spirit of the age; it got a lot of steam behind it. Mothers recruited mothers, etc., etc., but in fact the midwives were key, as usual.

Member of the audience: As usual, yes.

Mr Mike Wall: My recollection as a study father is probably similarly vague. Talking with my wife before I came here, she said she remembers having blood being taken from her at the GP, and being asked: 'Can we take a little bit more for this study?' So, you know, blood being taken, do you want to join? Her reaction immediately was 'yes', probably without knowing very much at all, but very quickly we understood the benefits, or potential benefits, of this project. Certainly the local nature, I can reinforce that. We moved into Bristol after our study child was conceived and it was a talking point that helped integrate us into the community that we were in. In terms of recruitment to the study, it was straightforward. For a little bit of effort on our part, we could see the potential benefits, perhaps not quite as Brian Pickering said to the 'health of the nation', but we thought we could contribute in our own little way. As a study father I can never remember thinking: 'Do I want to be involved with this?' It was always: 'There's a questionnaire, yes, I'm happy to do it.' So it was easy to say 'yes'.

Peckham: At the steering group meetings, we were always very impressed by the information we were shown on the feedback of information to parents and families, informing them about what was happening and the stage of the study. The focus on early feedback probably had a hugely important impact on recruitment. Would anyone like to say anything about how you decided on the materials you would use?

Golding: What, for the feedback?

Peckham: Yes, the feedback, because I think this was a very important part of the communication.

Hindi

स्वॉन मे रहने वाली सभी औरतों
जिनके बच्चों का जन्म अप्रैल १६६१
और अगस्त १६६२ के बीच होनेवला
होगा, की गर्भावस्था का अध्ययन
करने की यह एक नई उत्तेजिक
योजना है ।
इसमे भाग लेना दिलचस्प होगा । अधिक जानकरी के लिये
नीचे का परचा भरें व साथ मे दिये लिफाफे मे डालकर पोस्टकरें।

Figure 2: Card in Hindi introducing ALSPAC.

Golding: One of the staff that came forward, a bit like Sue Sadler, was Pam Holmes, who was married to a TV producer who did a programme about ALSPAC.[66] She watched it and said to him: 'Ooh, I'd like to be part of that.' So he introduced her and she had a background in publicity and public relations in general, so she was the person who designed our newsletters and posters and was particularly key in training staff on how to approach parents, because we had a whole network who were there to follow up if a mother hadn't returned a questionnaire. If, after a reminder or two, we still hadn't heard, they would ring up or call. Each of those interviewers had their own patch in the area and so got to know their participants very well. That was all part of what made it work.

Sadler: Following on from the interviews – one of the things interviewers did was to go to the scan clinics to interview the mothers, and in the process of that visit they would identify people who were not yet part of the study. That was another way of catching people who had been missed at the booking clinic, which is where, I think, most of the midwives would introduce the study to the

---

[66] We have not been able to find details of this particular programme, however, 'Children of the 90s' was featured on BBC2 *Close up West*, 3 February 1994. This was followed by a phone-in programme on local BBC radio programmes.

EXPECTING A BABY?

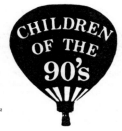

Dr. Jean Golding
Children of the Nineties
Institute of Child Health
24 Tyndall Avenue
Bristol, BS8 1BR

Figure 3: Expecting A Baby? Poster written in seven languages.

The First Two Months

A report from Dr. JEAN GOLDING

As we expected it has been two months of trial and error. Many of the things that we had piloted and showed to work have been put in motion and are now working superbly. Other details that were added somewhat at the last moment have worked less well and need to be worked out more fully.

It is only by getting the opinions and responses from all the health workers that we are able to identify any problems, and work out how to improve matters from the point of view both of the health professionals and, very importantly, of the mothers.

There have been two topics raised as particular problems so far. These have been miscarriage and blood sampling. The response to the miscarriage question is shown on the opposite page. The problems concerning blood samples will be discussed in our next issue. Please do keep us informed of all your problems so that we can address them.

Some of our difficulties have been because of the need to contact the mothers earlier in their pregnancy than we had done in our (very successful) pilot study. The logic is persuasive. After all, the embryo is likely to be most susceptible to the potential hazards or possible benefits of the environment during the very first months of pregnancy. The logistics, however, are a problem since ideally we need to contact women even before they see their community midwife.

To this end we have put up posters and have made cards available in numerous places including chemist shops, GP surgeries and Family Planning Clinics and we have had a lot of media coverage. Both cards and posters are available in seven ethnic minority languages. The idea is that the mother asks for a card which she fills in and posts to us in the reply-paid envelope in order to find out more about the study. We hope that women who have not already contacted us, will be given a card by their community midwives. Our last chance to make contact will be to use hospital computer lists of names and addresses. When we get the card we send out a brochure which outlines in some detail exactly what is going to happen within the survey and emphasises the freedom the woman has to opt in or out at any time. This is a mechanism that we have piloted fully, and shown that 95% of mothers find this wholly acceptable.

Once the mother has indicated her interest in the study, she will be sent a number of questionnaires. The first one is the Environment Questionnaire which ideally will reach her fairly early in pregnancy. Three more follow, and two others for her partner which she is free to hand to him, or not, as she chooses.

At delivery, no questions are asked of the mother, and the normal procedure of recording details is all that is required.

Subsequent contacts will use the same protocol and same design with mothers being contacted at 4-6 weeks postpartum, 6 months, 18 months and 3 years. All the information collected is designated the core information, and is separate from any special studies which may be added.

Within the ALSPAC programme, there are a number of people within Avon and elsewhere, who would like to mount special studies to look at particular aspects. For all such studies built onto the main ALSPAC core study, the parents who are invited to take part will get full details of the add-on study, and only those who offer to join will be included.

One of the proposed studies concerns the very detailed monitoring of a sub-sample of 120 parents' homes for all sorts of air pollutants like nitrogen dioxide, house dust mite debris and formaldehyde. These volunteer parents will have their air monitored over a 12 month period, and they will fill in detailed health diaries.

Not only do we have to present all the ideas for the study and documents to the three district health authority Ethical Committees, we also have our own survey ethical committee which advises on all aspects of the study. They make a careful judgement of the appropriateness or otherwise of the questions that we would like to ask, and weigh in balance any stress or distress that might occur. We also have a Parent Committee to advise on similar matters.

It is obvious to us from the responses we have had so far, how interested and excited mothers in Avon are, but one of our major problems is getting enough finance to do the survey adequately. We will shortly be asking local businesses in Avon if they would like to contribute in any way, and meanwhile we would be grateful for your ideas on how to raise money for this enormous but exciting project. Please feel free to ring our hotline (Bristol 256260) with any ideas or problems.

Jean Golding - 18 October 1990

ENCOURAGEMENT COMES FROM WOODSPRING

"May I wish you every success in this marvellous challenge which hopefully will open up many further avenues of research to unlock the mystery of why so many babies and children have such a wretched childhood through ill-health and no fault of their own".

Councillor J.C. Wiltshire
(Leader, Majority Group
Woodspring District Council).

Figure 4: ALSPAC Newsletter, Autumn 1990.

mothers. That was another way of doing it. We also had posters up at libraries and various other hospital waiting rooms, clinic waiting rooms, GP waiting rooms and so on, which may have attracted some people who wrote in, as many did from the outset. Incidentally, we also made a big effort to attract ethnic minority families, at least those where the mother was not English-speaking. We had little cards to introduce the study to the mothers printed in seven different Asian languages (see Figure 2).[67] I remember trying to find people who would do that translation from a group that I had been involved with before. I don't think we were hugely successful but I think it was very important that we did what we could. I made some visits to a local temple and a mosque and so on, trying to spread the word – we weren't very successful, but we tried.

Bowles: Again, in my notes and bits and pieces – I've mainly kept it for my son, as he grew up so he could see what he'd been involved in – this [holding up a document] was a newsletter for professionals and is dated autumn 1990. In it there is a report from Dr Jean Golding, The First Two Months (see Figure 4), and it says: '…we have put up posters and have made cards available in numerous places including chemist shops, GP surgeries and family planning clinics and we have had a lot of media coverage. Both cards and posters are available in seven ethnic minority languages [see Figures 2 and 3]. The idea is that the mother asks for a card which she fills in and posts to us… We hope that women who have not already contacted us, will be given a card by their community midwives. Our last chance to make contact will be to use hospital computer lists of names and addresses. When we get the card we send out a brochure which outlines in some detail exactly what is going to happen within the survey… Once the mother has indicated her interest in the study, she will be sent number of questionnaires.' So, yes, there were lots of ways in which everyone learned about this study at the time to become involved in it.

Stirrat: There was, of course, one important aspect of it that we must not forget and that is that quite a few women were recruited early in pregnancy and not all those pregnancies proceeded. Of course, even when they went to term, there

---

[67] Mrs Sue Sadler wrote: 'As far as I can remember, the cards were printed with text in Hindi, Urdu, Punjabi, Gujerati, Benghali, Chinese and Vietnamese. This was the only time we used other languages in printed material though we used the services of linkworkers for several years. The attempt to encourage non-English speaking ethnic minority women to join was not very successful. The head of the linkworkers, whom I knew, was herself from an immigrant family from India, said "our people are not ready to do this kind of altruistic work." She also felt that they would be unlikely to be prepared to divulge personal information to a linkworker, even if she was from the same community.' E-mail to Ms Caroline Overy, 8 December 2011.

were, unfortunately, some tragedies and some stillbirths. A huge amount of effort was put in to make absolutely certain that that was dealt with extremely sensitively, trying to balance the importance of information that might be obtained from such sad events – Jean might want to comment on that in a bit. These unfortunate women were facing this grief and tragedy, and we had to avoid forcing ourselves on them and adding to their grief. We had to be very careful to make sure that we didn't include someone in the continuing study who had unfortunately lost their child. I think it is important to mention that.

Golding: Yes, we did send mothers who had lost a child a special questionnaire, and in general, we got very favourable comments back. The sort of comments were: 'Nobody's been interested, but, you know, it has helped to write about what happened.' Many of those who lost a baby at the start of the study then enrolled with another pregnancy later, so we hadn't put them off.

Peckham: Very important.

Emond: One thing I would like to say, that I do regret about recruitment is that we didn't enrol fathers separately and in their own right. Because, over the years, with family reconstitution and so on, it's become extremely difficult to track men and to actually look at, not just their genetics, but also their influence on the family. I think it's very important for future cohorts, and I've already said this to Carol Dezateux[68] about the 2012 cohort, that men must be enrolled and followed up separately, and traced and tracked separately, because it's been very difficult unravelling ALSPAC further down the track to work out the influence of the man in the family. I know men are not very good at follow-up studies, but they need to be enrolled in their own right.

Peckham: Do you want to add anything to that, George, in terms of your current work?

Davey Smith: I would support that comment and we are currently attempting formal enrolment of the fathers and partners, but obviously it probably would have been simpler to do it earlier, and would have been more successful. But, of course, given the restrictions on funding, staffing, etc., it's difficult to do these things if the situation isn't pre-planned, as it will be in the 2012 cohort.

---

[68] Professor Carol Dezateux is director of the MRC Centre of Epidemiology for Child Health at UCL and leader of the scientific team responsible for the 2012 cohort; see note 41.

Golding: My memory – perhaps others can correct me – is that we deliberately decided not to enrol fathers and that was because we'd enrolled mothers, and we saw it as up to them to enrol their partner in the study if they wanted to. But it wasn't up to us. Obviously the Ethics Committee considered this, Elizabeth?

Mrs Elizabeth Mumford: I was secretary of the Ethics Committee at that time. I remember that we certainly considered the issue; it came up before the Ethics Committee, and we decided against it. I think we decided this because of the question in a lot of people's minds about the link with the issue of paternity and whether mothers might be upset at the thought that the samples would be used for paternity tracing. I think the figures we had at the time suggested that something between 5 and 30 per cent of children were going to be brought up by men who were not their natural fathers, but not all those men knew it. Would opening questions about biological samples in particular raise questions in people's minds and put them off the study entirely? I think, because of this, the Ethics Committee ruled against the idea. I don't know whether it was your suggestion that we should include fathers, but certainly somebody had proposed it and the Ethics Committee ruled against it.

Peckham: There had been a study done on paternity, I think, about that time, hadn't there, somewhere near Bristol, showing, I seem to remember, quite high rates of discordant partners.[69] I must say, I was very impressed early on about how valuable the creation of the Ethics Committee was. It was more than an ethics committee; it was more of an advisory committee, helping to make decisions about what could and couldn't be done, and how best to tackle problems. I thought that was very impressive and it had an important role both in terms of sample collections and questions asked. Now, Ian, you were involved in that aspect quite early on, weren't you?

Dr Ian Lister Cheese: I was a medical civil servant at the Department of Health at the time, and was captured by the interests of both Jean and Marcus separately, partly because I had policy responsibilities in child health, and also in genetics. At the end of the 1980s it seemed perfectly obvious that the right approach for the future was to study as carefully as one could the interaction of inborn and environmental factors in the development of children, a point made in the CMO's report *On the State of the Public Health for 1988*.[70] Yes, the Ethics

---

[69] For further discussion on non-paternity, see pages 36–38 and Appendix 5.

[70] Sir Donald Acheson (1926–2010) was Chief Medical Officer from 1983 to 1991; see Department of Health (1989): 73.

Committee was a remarkable idea. At that time local research ethics committees had a very wide remit; and it became clear that they couldn't give the deep and detailed and ongoing consideration to many often subtle proposals that the new ALSPAC Ethics Committee that eventually came into being, did. The committee never forgot that its first duty, its primary role, was to protect the participants of research. But it wasn't its only role and that is the point that Catherine has just made. It wasn't just an ethics committee, incidentally, it was an ethics and legal committee, and that too was important. Indeed, it reached further. It served as an ethics and legal and scientific appraisal committee, and was actually concerned to ensure that what was done was good science, but it also recognized that there was a tension between what might be the best science – in other words, what might be the fullest information that could be obtained, and the possible shortcomings and disadvantages of actually seeking that information. Some information might be potentially upsetting to parents; for example, where it touched on sexual health, sexual experience, questions of paternity, evidence of possible abuse and so on. There was a great deal of debate about the ways in which the study could be safeguarded and the willingness and keenness of participants maintained, not just at the outset, that was fairly easily done – you've seen the enthusiasm of parents from the beginning – but ongoing, year after year. Maintaining the reputation of ALSPAC was high among the concerns of the Ethics Committee. It had to preserve the reputation of the study. Yes, it did indeed do, and continues to do, all of these things.

Stirrat: Obviously there's a section on ethics later in the afternoon, but you want us to continue thinking of the Ethics and Law Committee, because I think this was one of David Baum's great contributions – just one, because he made quite a few. It was established very early and it was the Ethics and Law Committee, not just Ethics. Elizabeth is a lawyer, and it was chaired by a professor of law, Michael Furmston, who made a great contribution over the years.[71] That was extremely important because there were legal issues, opinions on which we didn't have to pay for. But that's a secondary matter – as a Scot I would remember that, but that's not the important thing. [Laughter] Of course we had epidemiologists, clinicians; we ultimately had an ethicist after Alastair

---

[71] Michael Furmston was appointed professor of law at the University of Bristol in 1978. He retired in 1998 and is currently emeritus professor and senior research fellow; since 2007 he has been professor of law at Singapore Management University.

Campbell was appointed to the chair of ethics in medicine in 1966.[72] Initially I pretended to be the ethicist on the committee. The committee was innovative in a variety of ways, one of which was that we had study mothers, including Ruth, as full members of the committee. That was extremely helpful. We also had a teacher. Ultimately, as the years progressed, we had fathers and young people, the progeny of ALSPAC, the 'Children of the 90s' themselves, now represented as full members. That was so, so important.

Among the rules that were set down, we had to get the balance right of being sufficiently prescriptive and proscriptive to protect the participants, as Ian has said, without producing such inflexible rules and regulations that further development was prevented. I think that was managed wonderfully well. I think it's a miracle that it was, but in fact, that's actually what happened. Obviously, we had to have very high levels of confidentiality and anonymity, and there was a 'golden rule' that those who collected data should in no way be involved in analysing it. There were, of course, occasions when some of the biological samples, for example, showed some results that were way out of the normal range, and we felt we had to have an avenue of going back to the individual. In general, the information people got was about how things were going in general in the study, not about their individual results. But there were occasions in which we felt we had to go back to the individual and we had to lay down the best rules we could, before this had been thought of by any other organization. We came up with the working rule that one had to have a strong indication of a condition that had a serious risk of harm for which there was a known remedy. We were also sure at that time, and still are, that we were not going to divulge genetic information. We got quite a lot of stick for that. The trump card they tried to play was autonomy, you know: 'it's our information, it's our right to get it',[73] but we were able to balance that, put autonomy in its proper place, with justice and with doing good and not doing harm. Given that the samples were not taken in clinical circumstances, didn't have clinical rigour and were for epidemiological studies, I think that worked quite well. In fact, it worked

---

[72] Professor Alastair Campbell is the director of the Centre for Biomedical Ethics at the National University of Singapore. Prior to this, he was professor of ethics in medicine in the Medical School of the University of Bristol and Director of its Centre for Ethics in Medicine. He attended the Witness Seminar 'Medical Ethics Education in Britain, 1963–1993', Reynolds and Tansey (2007), www.history.qmul.ac.uk/research/modbiomed/wellcome_witnesses/volume31/index.html (visited 31 January 2012).

[73] Professor Gordon Stirrat wrote: 'It was a few parents and also some lay members of ethics committees.' E-mail to Ms Caroline Overy, 12 February 2012.

so well that when the Biobank was being set up,[74] and Alistair Campbell, whose name I've mentioned already, was appointed to chair their Ethics Committee, he took the ALSPAC law and ethics rubric and criteria, and with some slight modification, applied them. That says a lot. Initially, of course, because the women and the participants were actually still 'patients', we had to put things to the local research ethics committees. That was not an entirely joyful experience: our relations with some of local research ethics committees (LREC) were fairly fraught, quite often due to a total misunderstanding of what it was that we were after, and that we were out of their comfort zone by a very long way. That created quite a lot of problems. We continued even although the participants were no longer 'patients' because at that time, interestingly enough, there was no research ethics committee within the university. That was established and the old habit of passing it onto LREC and their successors continued for a while, but certainly we now had this very clear relationship with the university research ethics committee. The Ethics and Law Committee was key to development and I think was a pathfinder in ethics and law for future studies.

Peckham: I was impressed by it and I think it had a great influence on how the study was run at the beginning. That's why I wanted to bring it up here, not just in the governance session later this afternoon.

Stirrat: We made Jean feel fairly uncomfortable from time to time, and therefore I think it was a success.[75]

Davey Smith: I was going to address your point about the non-paternity. In 1991 there was a high profile article in the *Lancet* by Sally MacIntyre and Anne Sooman on non-paternity and the issues of prenatal genetic screening, which did focus attention on this and issues around the ethics of genotyping mothers and fathers.[76] The article was very interesting because they said how non-paternity rates had taken on the air of urban folk tales, and they pointed out the uncertainty of many estimates. But even though they'd pointed out

---

[74] The UK Biobank, funded by the Wellcome Trust, the Medical Research Council, the Department of Health, the Scottish Executive and the Northwest Regional Development Agency was launched in Manchester in 2006 to gather biological samples and medical and lifestyle data from 500 000 people aged 40 to 69. It is a long-term research programme to create a national database to improve prevention, diagnosis and treatment of serious illness. See, for example, Elliott and Peakman (2008).

[75] Professor Gordon Stirrat added an exclamation mark and noted that 'this is meant affectionately, of course'. Note on draft transcript, 6 September 2011.

[76] MacIntyre and Sooman (1991).

that these were urban myths, that paper ended up getting quoted by some as the source of the famous 10 per cent figure, which it was actually a critique of. There were two other things: one is the importance, I think, of recruiting parent figures, not saying you're recruiting them because they are the biological mother or biological father, but because they are parent figures, which is certainly something we're attempting to do now when enrolling father figures in the study. But the message is quite difficult to convey, particularly because in a study that is set up about antenatal events, the parent figures are filling out questionnaires, which all appear to be about them being parents. One of the ALSPAC fathers was visiting me for some other reason, but then said in the lift that he was an ALSPAC dad and he'd dropped in to a clinic – we have drop-in clinics where dads are enrolled and blood samples taken at the moment – and I said that he was going to be invited for clinical examination. He was rather surprised at that because he thought we were only interested in the dads as a source of DNA. We try to say that the interest is in the health of the men, and that we are using all the information that has been collected over 20 years to examine this. ALSPAC is an incredibly valuable resource for looking at the dads, along with the mothers, in their own right, not just as the parents of the index child in ALSPAC. The last thing, which Marcus might talk about, is that I think it would also be fair to say that 20 years ago there was less interest in fathers in terms of having biological influences on offspring. There was a huge literature on maternal effects, but there was a rather limited literature on paternal effects in the genetic field. Interest in this has grown over the past 20 years.[77]

Pembrey: Yes. Obviously there were various scientific reasons why we might want to have samples from the fathers and this was relevant to the enrolling of fathers to begin with. We can cover those in the section on the genetics, but this question of what's called non-paternity – unexpected paternity is the right phrase. It just happens that I'm responsible for the quote of 5 per cent. I can guarantee the source of this information, it is the Government's figure in *Hansard*.[78] I don't think it's been quoted since. Five per cent (and at least 5 per cent) was what was quoted by Lord MacKay of Clashfern when the Lords were concerned about birth certificates and gamete donation, sperm and egg donation, during the lead up to the first Human Fertilisation and Embryology

---

[77] See, for example, Pembrey *et al.* (2006).

[78] Human Fertilisation and Embryology Bill [H.L.] Lords *Hansard;* Column 1317, HL Deb, 13 February 1990, vol 515, cols 1317–18; Lord MacKay of Clashfern was Lord Chancellor (1987–97); see Appendix 5 for part of his speech.

Bill in 1990. Many Lords were saying that surely the birth certificate defined who the biological father was, and we had to disabuse them of the fact. So Lord MacKay wanted a figure. It just happened, as Ian Lister Cheese will know, that I had been appointed in the previous year as the consultant advisor in genetics to the Chief Medical Officer and so it was my lot to sort this out, which I can assure you I did in a very scientifically rigorous way.[79] There was some background to paternity testing at the time, but this wasn't, of course, why we were interested in enrolling fathers into ALSPAC. I absolutely take the point that George says, that it was the father as a person that we were interested in.

Peckham: The changing attitude to the role of fathers is interesting. Are there any questions that you didn't ask that you regretted later or wished you had? Is there any area that you regretted you didn't cover, with hindsight?

Golding: With hindsight, I would have loved to have sent questionnaires to the grandparents, because that's the generation that is very important regarding the parents of our study children, and it would have been good to capture them before they dropped off more than they had already. With work that Marcus and I are doing, the intergenerational effects of traumas and such things that happen during one's upbringing can be passed down the generations, and that would have been good to capture.[80] There is a biological sample I would have liked to capture too, which Jon Pollock piloted, and we decided we just didn't have the money for, and that was breast milk. I'm sure there are lots of other things, but that's today's thought.

Peckham: So what were the samples you collected in pregnancy? You collected the placentas.

Golding: We collected several maternal bloods and urines during pregnancy, the placentas, the umbilical cord tissue and cord blood.

Peckham: We'll be talking about those later. Are there any other questions or issues that we need to highlight in the areas that we've already discussed?

---

[79] Professor Marcus Pembrey wrote: 'In the last few decades of the twentieth century, an experienced practitioner in each of the main medical disciplines was appointed to advise the Chief Medical Officer on a relatively ad hoc basis. A consultant advisor in genetics was established in 1972 (Cedric Carter), Rodney Harris followed him and I was the third (1989–98)'. E-mail to Ms Caroline Overy, 1 January 2012.

[80] See, for example, Pembrey *et al.* (2006).

Emond: The other reflection I'd like to make is about the issue of consent, because when consenting for a longitudinal study you've really got to try to anticipate what the consent parameters, the ethical parameters, will be in the future. It's very difficult. In retrospect, the consent we got from the mothers for engagement in ALSPAC was fine at the time, but it's proved tricky further down the track as expectations on consent have got greater. So, for example, we're re-consenting the young people for record linkage, whereas when the mothers were pregnant we gained opt-out consent for access to medical records. It's not the same thing. That is a reflection for future cohorts, to try to think slightly longitudinally about consent and what it could mean in the future, not the standard at the moment. You can bet your bottom dollar it will change.

Peckham: In the 1958 cohort in the early phase, no consent was sought. Information was collected by health visitors who were already visiting the families. It merely formalized their activities and they felt very much part of the study. It becomes more difficult when the child becomes an adult and consent is sought from them rather than the mother.

Sadler: There is something we've touched on, particularly talking about ethics and recruitment and so on, but I'd like to mention it in a different way, and that is the way we treated our families. I should have said something about it when talking about recruiting staff. I went on recruiting many people for the rest of my time in ALSPAC, and the thing I was always looking for first was the right person, one who had the warmth, the sensitivity, the interest and the ability to make a rapport – that was the word, you know – to make a rapport quickly with the families, who had the interest of the family very much at heart. That sort of ethos of the study which came originally from Jean, I think, and also came from the Ethics Committee. I want to read you a paragraph, if I may, of what I used to say, and which we had to bring up in our induction of staff. It wasn't only me who did that, it was other team members, but it went:

> We aim to collect the maximum number of repeatable data on every child and we aim to make every child's and every family's experience of their visit positive. When there is a potential conflict between these two, the child's need comes first. So if the child has reservations that you cannot readily overcome, or is experiencing pain or distress, and wants you to stop, you do. The child is in charge. That applies even when the parent is telling you to go ahead, or the child not to make a fuss. The trick is to handle the situation so that both feel good about it. The danger of not doing so is obvious: we may do harm to the child, the

family may not come back, they may tell their friends and peers. We are a longitudinal study: we rely on having repeat measures over time and on maximizing numbers.[81]

I think that, along with everything we did, that was an example of the way we dealt with the families and the respect and gratitude that we had, and the way we kept it longitudinal. It was practical as well as caring.

Peckham: That was a nice statement.

Bowles: Respect for the participants is key in explaining why people have remained interested in the study. Reading back through my records as well, I remember taking part in different aspects of the science; so putting the test tubes outside the window, having to record the temperature of the room, that was actually taking part in science.[82] I think lots of people don't have that opportunity. For future studies, I think giving something for the individuals to do is also quite good in maintaining interest. How reliable that is is a different matter, but people were actually taking part in the science. A lot of people that I spoke to, the other mothers, at one point were quite upset to hear that the study might stop because of the lack of funding, whilst recognizing how valuable all the science was.

Peckham: And how much do the children appreciate it now? That's obviously very important, isn't it?

Bowles: Throughout all the various Focus Clinics, my son was involved in a Focus Clinic right from the start, each time they went they were given different, interesting things to do. They may have been given a picture to take home with them of some interesting aspect of their body, you know, so a retinal image or something, that they would never have the opportunity to see anywhere else. They could have any of the bone scans that had been done, get an image of that, for example (see Figure 5). All of those sorts of things helped to maintain the interest for the children who have been involved, but also the parents as well. As I say, taking part in the science.

Wall: Can I just say, as a study father, I think my son always enjoyed going to the annual or the study days, and I certainly remember him describing it as a 'fun day', and I'd reinforce that that was really important in retaining his interest in the study over the longer term.

---

[81] Written by Mrs Sue Sadler for use by the team leaders in the training of new staff.

[82] For the letter of instructions for the ALSPAC air study, see Appendix 6.

Total Body Bone Density

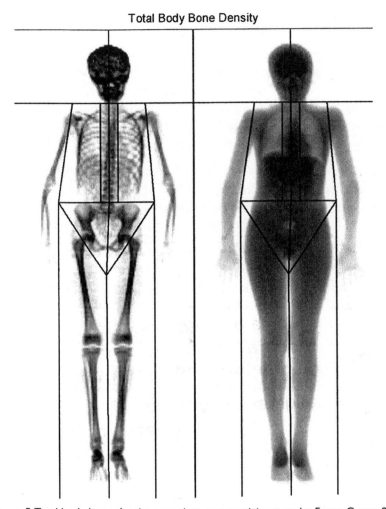

Figure 5: Total body bone density scan given to a participant at the Focus Group 9+.

Stirrat: There were also parties and that sort of thing for them, and Jean can comment further on that. There was good fun to be had. But when they became teenagers, a Teenage Advisory Panel was set up of the young people, and it was tremendous to be involved with them, it really was.[83] They were engaged and interested, and asked some very difficult questions. Three of them then came and sat in on the Ethics and Law Committee for a while before becoming full members. They really asked some very, very hard questions and it was very

---

[83] For details of the Teenage Advisory Panel, see Appendix 7.

important that they were not patronized.[84] I think we had a little bit of difficulty with that to begin with and some of them were a little bit upset about that. I think we ultimately got that right and their inclusion was a valuable innovation. It was not just public relations, it was much more fundamental and important than that. It involved them in the study and kept them coming. Although, of course, young men are not so amenable to continuing in this study perhaps as young women and there was a bit more fall off among the former.[85] So that's another very positive aspect: the Teenage Advisory Panel was really very good.

Peckham: It seems to me that a lot of what has been said is very much due to the fact that it is a local study, there is a total buying-in by the community. I think this would have been much more problematic if the cohort had been recruited across the whole country; based on your experience it will be very interesting to see how these issues are addressed in the new cohort.

Golding: I think one of the interesting things will be to see whether the 'Children of the 90s', the children in ALSPAC, have had an influence on what people decide to do in terms of the A-levels they take; the university courses they do, whether it's related to some of the things we have studied with them, and whether that's different from the cohorts that went before or come after, which should be easy to do, actually.

Davey Smith: Whilst it doesn't really relate to what Jean said, one issue is, that it's been found that some people who would have been eligible to be recruited into 'Children in the 90s' but for various reasons weren't, and we are now obviously trying to get permission for record linkage, etc. If we do get permission it will actually be possible, in an almost experimental way, to see the differences between those who were recruited and those who weren't.

Peckham: I would like to start with the collection of the samples, because I think that this study was unique in that it did collect placenta samples. You were involved, weren't you, Sue, in the collection of the cord bloods, the placenta, antenatal samples and blood samples?

---

[84] Professor Gordon Stirrat wrote: 'When you have a group of senior academics and very experienced lay people talking about important matters affecting the study it took some time to find the right balance between talking above the heads of the young people and being thought to be talking down to them.' E-mail to Ms Caroline Overy, 11 December 2011.

[85] Professor Gordon Stirrat wrote: 'Between the ages of 16–18 years, the number of girls still participating was 57 per cent and boys 42 per cent.' E-mail to Ms Caroline Overy, 20 December 2011.

Sadler: Yes, only in the sense that I was one of, and a very, very junior member of, the biological samples team.

Peckham: You will remember it well then. [Laughter]

Sadler: I was the gofer, I think.

Peckham: You can tell the truth. [Laughter]

Sadler: I've had a chance to look over the minutes again, thanks to Yasmin and Jean, but my memory is that the two main problems were whether we got the samples from all the women and from all the different hospitals, and when we got them what on earth were we going to do with them? In the sense that there simply wasn't the space to store these things. The -20°C space for the urines and the -70°C, as we then had to have for the bloods.[86] The cost of providing this space was, of course, beyond us at the time, wasn't it, team? One or two things do come back to me, and I think they are quite important: one is the way we had to work. I often had to go around talking to midwives in different hospitals and clinics, and that reminds me of just how much these midwives did for the study. For heaven's sake, they had a job to do, their concern was for the mothers and their babies, and that's a full-time business, but they were still willing to find the time to fill extra tubes and consult the mother to get her agreement, and talk to her about the placenta, record her details and so on and so on – and, to do it properly. We had problems with some areas where the midwives were getting it wrong, or they hadn't got the right tubes or what have you, but basically they were willing to do it, the vast majority of them, and I think that's extraordinary. It came from the top: the midwife managers were prepared to help, and obviously Gordon Stirrat had a huge influence over that. It was typical of the goodwill that this study attracted, and the generosity. When it came to spaces in freezers and so on, I remember Professor Mott[87] offering part of his -70°C freezer, for example. Other people offered a bit of their lab space. Things over and above what people needed to do.

Peckham: The mothers were quite happy about the samples being taken? There was no concern there? Did they know what they were for?

---

[86] -70°C is the optimal temperature to store samples to avoid degradation and in terms of future stability; see, for example, Elliott and Peakman (2008).

[87] Martin V Mott, emeritus professor of paediatric oncology.

Sadler: Well, I can only imagine that some of them must not have done because what we were getting was, if not samples from all the births, certainly the very large majority of them, and I suspect that some of those were not actually people who were enrolled. Jean will probably correct me if I'm wrong.

Golding: What we did at birth was to ask the midwives at delivery to save the placentas, regardless of whether the mother was part of 'Children of the 90s' or not. We would sort it out later. We would only analyse their placentas or the cord blood if we had their written permission, but at the time we wouldn't know, and you couldn't get that sorted out in time. So that when the mothers enrolled in pregnancy, they had a brochure that described that we would be collecting placentas and cord blood, but we wouldn't touch them until we had their signed permission. The signed permission would have been got during pregnancy wherever possible. We paid some of our staff to go into the ultrasound clinics that did scans at 18 weeks' or 16 weeks' gestation. Our staff were there to chat up the mothers and ask if they would consent to their biological samples being analysed. So, that was an important part of the antenatal process. If we hadn't got permission or hadn't had time to contact them, then we would try and contact them later, but I think that was more by post than anything else. But it was the personal discussion that was important, but midwives couldn't do that at the time of delivery when all sorts of clinical things were happening.

Stirrat: Of course, there's an area here that is not mentioned: a group of unsung heroes, because there was the collection of data as well, extracted from the case notes, with permission. This group of wonderful nurses and midwives – I think Sue could probably talk about them[88] – did a tremendous job of trying to understand my handwriting, for example, and trying to collect the relevant data from the case notes. That was extremely important as one aspect of collection.

Golding: Gordon, that's still going on. We're still trying to translate you. [Laughter]

Peckham: That was data on the pregnancy complications?

Stirrat: The data on each of the indexed pregnancies of the mothers, yes.

---

[88] Professor Gordon Stirrat wrote: 'On discussion I have ascertained that Sue Sadler was not involved in the abstraction of obstetric data from medical records. Trudy Goodenough initially supervised the team who were already in place having just finished data abstraction for the Vitamin K and "Cancer in Childhood" study (appointed and trained by Karen Birmingham). When Karen returned from a year abroad, she took over the supervision of the team and continued in that role for a decade or so.' E-mail to Ms Caroline Overy, 20 December 2011.

Peckham: That's still being analysed at the moment?

Golding: No, it's one of the things we stopped doing when we ran out of money, and we've only done it when we've had the money to do it, unlike everything else. We had thought that the computer system in each of the big maternity hospitals was going to give us the data that we wanted, and we did a pilot study, and it was basically rubbish. So we had to, and are still having to, extract the information from the medical records. Medical records can be six inches thick; it's not a trivial exercise.

Peckham: No, I know it's not.

Golding: So we have had trained staff that Karen Birmingham supervised for quite a long time, and extracted data on 8 000 of our 13 000, nearly 14 000, deliveries. There are 5 500 left to do, and they will be destroyed in 2015, so we're trying hard to get the money to do that. That's rather critical to looking at factors operating during pregnancy that are clinically relevant; the sort of medication used, etc.

Peckham: What about the documentation that went with the placentas?

Golding: There wasn't any documentation. [Laughs] It depended on which hospital; the placentas were put into formalin with an identifying label, to be sorted out. The cord blood similarly; there was a sample that was kept in a fridge which was for clinical purposes, and retrieved when it was no longer needed, and then an extra sample taken if we were lucky.

Dr Sue Ring: I'm now head of the ALSPAC laboratories, and I want to say that I wasn't around when all the samples were collected, but I think that there was a lot of work going on behind the scenes in the lab that people aren't mentioning. The documentation we have in the lab is very good. We have dates that samples were collected, dates that they were aliquoted and frozen down; and it wasn't just a case of a sample being taken and put in a fridge.

Peckham: Alan, you were telling me a story earlier about the placentas. I wonder if you could tell us all?

Emond: It was common practice, but not widely known, that maternity hospitals used to sell placentas for cosmetics.[89] It was traditionally viewed by the midwives as a bit of a perk, and the money that was gained, I think in most hospitals,

---

[89] Professor Emond wrote: 'The placenta is a source of oestrogen, which is used in anti-ageing skin creams; there are occasional newspaper articles about this practice, see, for example, Sawyer (2008).' E-mail to Ms Caroline Overy, 2 February 2012.

went into what was effectively a slush fund for midwives to use. It was only a small amount of money per placenta and I suspect the cosmetic companies made huge profits out of it. The important thing was that most women who delivered didn't know that that was going to happen, and the hospitals were, in my view, unethical in not telling them. So when ALSPAC came along and wanted to take the placentas away, this was a potential barrier to the midwives' participation, so Jean found a solution, as you might imagine. [Laughter]

Golding: Extra costs.

Emond: I'm not sure how it was funded, but we managed to pay 50p per placenta.

Peckham: So what happened to the placentas that they kept, that you didn't want?

Golding: We didn't sort them; we kept all the placentas.

Peckham: Even though they weren't study placentas?

Golding: We didn't know that they weren't study placentas for a while.

Peckham: So you had to store all the placentas?

Golding: Most of them were. I mean, we were enrolling 80+ per cent of all pregnancies.

Pembrey: Can I just come back to the question that Sue Ring had asked: what actually happened with these samples? Obviously leading up to the deliveries there was a lot of discussion about what samples needed to be collected, but they went into the NHS system. Charles Pennock was the head of biochemistry or chemical pathology,[90] and they got stored there and properly labelled in various ways. For example, I can talk about the sample that was there for DNA extraction: there was no way the Law and Ethics Committee would allow us to extract the DNA until the consents from the mothers for the analysis had been computer linked with the samples. So there was quite a lag, a year or two or more probably, between the samples being carefully collected and the consents being linked to them and their having their final resting place, as it were, ready for use. One thing I would like to know beyond just the blood samples and placenta; what about the tooth fairy and things like that? I've always wondered who organized that?

---

[90] Dr Charles Pennock worked for the Bristol and Weston Health Authority, becoming a consultant in paediatric chemical pathology; in 1972 he was appointed senior lecturer in child health at the University of Bristol.

Sadler: We sent letters out to parents about the tooth fairy, and then we sent out packages for them to send the teeth in to us. Kaija Turvey was responsible, I think, for logging the teeth in when they arrived.

Golding: We then sent back a badge at great expense [Laughter] to thank the child. I heard from another cohort study that they'd found the tooth fairy a great problem politically; I think it was the Christchurch New Zealand study that found that in trying to be the tooth fairy by giving money for the tooth, they were giving more money than many of the normal mothers in their study would have actually paid – this was seen as a disaster from their point of view.[91] Conversely, the alternative, if you paid less, would have been a disaster. So we decided on financial grounds too, that we certainly wouldn't pay, we would give a badge.

Sadler: We did have the newsletter didn't we, to help? We had articles in there and pictures of the tooth fairy, our tooth fairy, which was Kaija (see Figure 6), to encourage the children to understand what it was being done for as well.[92]

Miss Karen Birmingham: I was also extremely junior at the start of ALSPAC, but one thing I was asked to do, as I had a nursing background, was to pilot some of the biological samples.[93] One which I have just remembered was that I had to go to get antenatal urine from two GP practices. Two GP practices in rather deprived areas of Bristol were chosen, and we arranged to go along. I don't know, I have asked Elizabeth and she says she doesn't remember this going through the Ethics Committee, but, I sat in the treatment room sluice and the midwives would bring me these samples of urine, and I would put a number on them and take them back to ALSPAC. I wasn't quite sure what was happening to them but I gather they were analysed for, among other things, illicit drugs, and I think that cannabis came out quite high, higher than expected. The next

---

[91] See Fergusson *et al.* (1989). The Christchurch Health and Development Study tooth fairy inflated the going-rate for teeth by 150 per cent from 20 cents to 50 cents; see David Fergusson's speech: The Christchurch Health and Development Study, at /www.parliament.nsw.gov.au/prod/parlment/committee. nsf/0/c33c46f2a40e4e0cca256c2a0006a7fe/$FILE/The%20Development%20of%20Wellbeing%20 in%20Children%20Part%202%20Fergusson.pdf, 19–20 (visited 11 January 2012).

[92] Funded by the National Asthma Campaign, studies carried out on children's two top front teeth, which begin to develop before birth, showed that they contained a detailed record of pre-birth exposure to trace elements and minerals; see www.bristol.ac.uk/alspac/documents/tooth-fairy.pdf (visited 4 October 2011).

[93] Miss Karen Birmingham wrote: 'Only antenatal urine samples were collected in this particular example. I also piloted the collection of cord blood for cell line transformation and placentas but this is not relevant in this context.' E-mail to Ms Caroline Overy, 9 December 2011.

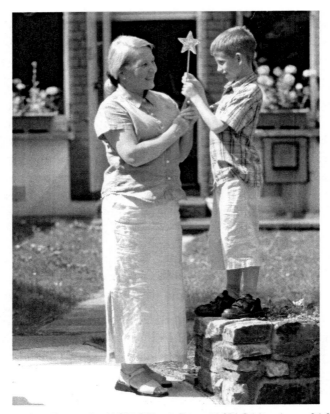

Figure 6: Kaija Turvey, the ALSPAC Tooth Fairy, ALSPAC Newsletter 26 2003.

thing I knew, as a very junior member of staff, was a consultant obstetrician ringing me up and saying he wanted the names of all these mothers. I said, 'Well, they were collected anonymously so I'm afraid I can't give them.' 'Don't give me that! I shall go to Jean Golding and find them.' A lot of pressure was put on me. They were anonymous, thank goodness, but I did think that was, well, I was very glad they were anonymous, because he was quite threatening in order to get it, because he was responsible for these people's care; they were his patients and he needed to know who they were.

Peckham: Did the mothers know what the urines were being tested for? Now you would have to get consent to do this.

Birmingham: Absolutely.

Golding: This wasn't an ALSPAC sample. This was a pilot to see what the problems were likely to be. It was a pilot.

Peckham: It was still without consent?

Golding: Yes.

Peckham: You couldn't do that now without consent. We had problems with the collection of oral fluids in the Millennium cohort.[94] You might not know who they are, but you still need consent to collect the samples. No doubt that would have gone through your Ethics Committee?

Birmingham: I don't think it did go through the Ethics Committee. I think it happened before the Ethics Committee was set up. It was definitely a pilot to see how easy or difficult it was to get hold of urine from the GP practices. One other thing, because I was in charge, for quite a long time, of supervising the midwives collecting data from medical records, and talking about handwriting: there was one midwife whose handwriting we all recognized; she was very well known. The blood pressures antenatally for every woman she ever took blood pressure from was 120/70. [Laughter]

Dr Richard Jones: I worked in the labs at ALSPAC for a while. Before we lose sight of the neonatal cord samples, I want to underline what a brilliant opportunity birth is for sample collection. You never get as much blood from the infant again for many years. My second observation is that the quality of those samples, certainly in ALSPAC, was very good, whereas a lot of earlier collections from the mother were compromised from the difficult situations in which they were collected by ALSPAC.

Peckham: A lot of studies have had difficulties in collecting cord samples because you cannot predict when women will deliver and there are often locum midwives on duty and you miss your samples.[95]

---

[94] Professor Catherine Peckham wrote: 'Consent was obtained from the parent for the collection of oral fluids in the Millennium cohort. The recording of this consent is essential as problems arose when samples were sent to the lab and tested but subsequent data linkage did not record consent in all cases.' E-mail to Ms Caroline Overy, 6 February 2012. For the collection of oral fluid samples, see Bartington *et al.* (2009).

[95] Professor Catherine Peckham wrote: '... there are often locum midwives on duty who have not been trained to take the samples correctly or are not aware of the protocol and consent. We had experience of this in a large prospective study of CMV infection in pregnancy and had to abandon this.' E-mail to Ms Caroline Overy, 6 February 2012. The NHS Cord Blood Bank for voluntary donations of cord blood after birth opened in London in November 2011, www.nhsbt.nhs.uk/cordblood/index.asp (visited 11 January 2012). See also Ong *et al.* (1999).

Jones: ALSPAC did it, and birth is an absolute golden opportunity. It's one of the major arguments, from a biological point of view, for having recruitment before birth. Clearly you won't get anything decent retrospectively from that time point. If you wanted to establish a DNA collection, with the benefit of hindsight again, cord bloods would have been a perfect opportunity both in terms of the quality of the sample and the coverage that is potentially there. Coverage is far, far more difficult in later stages.[96]

Stirrat: You asked Jean about missed opportunities and in fact Marcus has referred to a visit to Porton Down. A group of us went and that was the golden opportunity for establishing a DNA collection from cord bloods, because that's what was planned. If you're looking at one of the things that was a major disappointment and in fact, ultimately, has probably cost a great deal more and produced a great deal less information on DNA, it was the turning down of the request to actually immortalize these cell lines from umbilical cords.[97] That was a missed opportunity which can never be repeated.

Peckham: That's important to document.

Golding: Charles Pennock[98] didn't actually believe that there was much point in collecting these biological samples. He was facilitating it, but thought nobody was ever going to want to do anything with them; it was a waste of time, a waste of money, and at the end of a meeting he used to say: 'I'm ALSPACed', which meant, you know, just too much. However, the fact that he kept doing it and the data is in such a good state is, I think, amazing.

Ring: I want to pick up on Gordon's comment there that it was a missed opportunity with the cord bloods and not getting cell lines. In retrospect now, I don't think that's true. Some of the epigenetics projects that we're currently working on are dependent on using DNA extracted from the white cells that

---

[96] See, for example, Moise (2005).

[97] Professor Gordon Stirrat wrote: 'In fact Porton Down did not turn down the request; indeed they were eager to be involved in the creation of cell lines. Unfortunately (and in my opinion short-sightedly) none of the funding bodies was prepared to fund this initiative.' E-mail to Ms Caroline Overy, 20 December 2011.

[98] See note 90.

were not transformed.[99] Therefore the samples that were collected are very, very useful for epigenetic projects and if we hadn't had those samples, that would have been a missed opportunity now.

Peckham: So there has been a gain and a loss.

Jones: Did you mean, Sue, the ability to compare the DNA collected at birth with DNA collected later?

Ring: Yes, exactly, which is what we are now doing.

Peckham: Can you distinguish easily between maternal DNA and child DNA? I mean, when you have cord samples? Is that not sometimes a problem?

Ring: I don't think it really is a problem. We did some studies very early on where we were looking at the samples from boys to see if any had evidence of two X chromosomes, and it was a small number, less than 1 per cent.

Golding: One thing that we haven't covered is collecting the samples from the children themselves, because that was very important. And we had this 10 per cent sample of Children in Focus that we took heel prick samples from. Now heel prick samples are actually very painful …[100]

Peckham: It depends on the age, doesn't it?

Golding: I think even if you're a four-month-old it is painful. When we started using venepuncture, we used an anaesthetic cream and that worked much better, and was much less of a hassle and less painful for the child, and the parent.[101]

---

[99] Epigenetics is the study of heritable changes in gene expression that do not involve changes in DNA sequence; see notes 114 and 138. Dr Sue Ring wrote: 'We currently have funding (ARIES project funded by the Biotechnology and Biological Sciences Research Council (BBSRC)) to obtain epigenetic data (Illumina HumanMethylation450 BeadChip) on serial samples for 1000 mother-child pairs using DNA extracted from blood taken from the children at birth (cord blood), 7 years and 15–17 years and from their mothers during pregnancy and 15 to 17 years later. The first paper related to this work is Relton *et al.* (2012).' E-mail to Ms Caroline Overy, 30 January 2012.

[100] On heel pricks, see, for example, Owens and Todt (1984); Slater *et al.* (2006). For an ALSPAC 'Children in Focus' study using the heel prick, see Emond *et al.* (1996).

[101] For heel prick vs venepuncture, see, for example, Shah *et al.* (1997); Shah and Ohlsson (2007).

So blood samples were possible, the Ethics Committee approved of them, and we've collected other biological samples from the children as well. Some of the offspring give blood every time they come nowadays.[102]

Peckham: That's very interesting. Marcus, you were on the Ethics Committee of the British Paediatric Association (BPA), as it was then,[103] when it looked at ethics in research in children and concluded that taking a blood sample from a normal child was invasive and not ethical.[104]

Pembrey: Yes. It was indeed.

Peckham: I remember the debates that went on around this issue.

Pembrey: It was indeed and I absolutely want to reiterate my admiration for the system they [ALSPAC] had for taking venepunctures from children. This was probably the first time EMLA cream[105] was used in epidemiological scale studies. Of course, in hospital EMLA cream, the anaesthetic cream, got a slightly bad reputation. The child usually had it put on for too short a time, and it was clearly linked psychologically with having the needle, whereas the way they sorted it out in the clinic for ALSPAC was absolutely admirable, you know. The magic cream would be put on and then they would be doing all sorts of other things and exactly three quarters of an hour later, or whatever it was, they then came back.[106] I understand that more often than not the toddlers cried because the video of *Postman Pat* had been turned off than during the venepuncture, so it was brilliant.

---

[102] Blood, hair and urine were collected at the 15+ and 17+ clinics. Dr Larisa Duffy, head of fieldwork for ALSPAC, wrote: 'There is not currently a clinic for study children but there is a plan to have a sweep in 2014/15. Also there is a number of sub-studies taking place currently but they involve a small subset of the cohort (either by genotype or phenotype) and often do not include the blood sample.' E-mail to Ms Caroline Overy, 8 March 2012.

[103] Now the Royal College of Paediatrics and Child Health; it received Royal College status in 1996.

[104] Professor Marcus Pembrey supplied the following reference: 'LOW risk procedures that cause brief pain or tenderness, and small bruises or scars. Many children fear needles and for them LOW rather than MINIMAL risks are often incurred by injections or venepuncture… It would be unethical to submit child subjects to more than MINIMAL risk when the procedure offers no benefit to them, or only a slight or very uncertain one.' British Paediatric Association (1992): 4.' E-mail to Ms Caroline Overy, 1 January 2012.

[105] EMLA®, a registered trademark of APP Pharmaceuticals, is a local anaesthetic (an abbreviation for Eutectic Mixture of Local Anesthetics), containing 2.5% lidocaine (lignocaine) and 2.5% prilocaine.

[106] On the use of EMLA cream, see, for example, Lander *et al.* (1996); Rogers and Ostrow (2004).

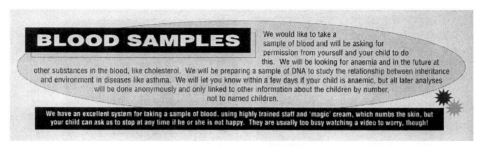

Figure 7: Information on blood sampling from the Focus@7 leaflet.

Peckham: What age were these children?

Sadler: We started at age two, I think. It was either two or two-and-a-half, wasn't it, Jean? Two-and-a-half, we started – I've got a picture somewhere here (see Figure 8) – 31 months, yes. Two and a half. Exactly as Marcus said, the venepunctures worked brilliantly. We took a lot of trouble getting it right, though. We had a play leader from the hospital to talk about playing with the children, distracting them during the procedure. We had these wonderful videos: *Postman Pat* was the first one we used, because they got older as we went on. We also took a lot of trouble over the technique. We ended up using Sarstedt Monovettes,[107] which I don't think were much used in the hospitals, but with butterflies.[108] We had the rep down and one of his assistants thoroughly trained the staff in using them because I don't think many of them had actually used them before. We very, very rarely used a syringe. It was exceptional if one of the people used a syringe. The other thing is, we chose our blood takers with enormous care. For many, many years these were very experienced paediatric phlebotomists; we only used them for most of the time I was there. Towards the end of my time, which was in 2008, we had spent a couple of years using them to train up one or two of the staff that were suitable, were keen and interested to do it, and several of them became also extremely good phlebotomists. Phlebotomy in children is a real art: you really need people who are expert at it, and we had a team who could get blood out of anything, I swear. They were absolutely brilliant and it was so rare for a child to be in the least bit bothered.

---

[107] The Sarstedt S-Monovette® is a closed blood collection system that collects blood using either the aspiration or vacuum principle of collection.

[108] Mrs Sue Sadler wrote: '… phlebotomists at the time …were used to using syringes. Ours had to be trained to use the Monovettes, but once practised with them and the butterfly needles, they found them much simpler to use on small children. We used EMLA cream too, put on an hour in advance.' E-mail to Ms Caroline Overy, 8 December 2011.

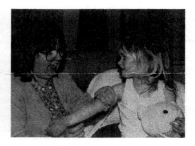

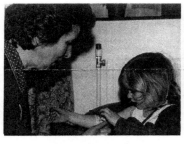

1. Putting on the 'magic cream'

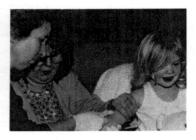

2. The cream comes off after an hour

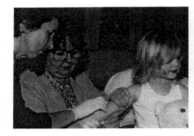

3. We find a vein. Zoe watches Postman Pat

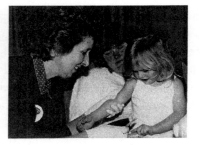

4. The needle goes in. Zoe doesn't notice

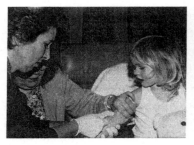

5. The sample is taken. "Mmm...that's interesting".

6. Now, which plaster? "The Flintstones please".

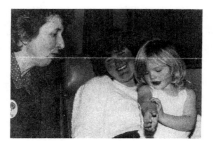

7. All finished. Well done Zoe, mum and the staff!

Figure 8: Taking blood at the 2½ year clinic.

It's very sad that subsequently that team were not taken on again when things changed at the clinics. It's a great grief to me that they were lost as a whole, as a group. Because it was felt important that people were able to do blood-taking as well as this, that and the other. But these highly qualified people were absolutely brilliant and trained some other people to be as good.

Peckham: Was this taken up in the Ethics Committee, because this would have been quite interesting?

Mumford: Yes, the Ethics Committee was acutely aware of what was going on at the British Paediatric Association.[109] Various other regulatory bodies had also issued guidance.[110] There was quite a controversy at the time.[111] There was a lot of discussion about terminology in an attempt to set the appropriate standard: which words to use. People talked of 'minimal risk' versus 'negligible risk'. What we did was to go along and watch. We were invited and so we went and observed blood being taken with real interest. I was certainly one of those who was not convinced that having blood taken was not going to be distressing for the child. That was the benchmark that we had decided to use: would it cause distress for the children? When we left, I was convinced, as was, I think, everybody else on the committee: we saw the whole procedure and we felt that it was genuinely not causing distress. The children appeared relaxed; they appeared happy as they sat watching the video and that convinced us that we could give ethical approval for the venepuncture. The other thing that we did, when the children were aged four or five, was to start allowing them to make the decision themselves whether they were going to give blood. This was no longer purely a parental decision. At that age, children are clearly not old enough to give consent in the legal sense, but we allowed them to say 'yes' or 'no', in a meaningful way, that

---

[109] British Paediatric Association (1992); see note 103.

[110] For example, Royal College of Physicians (1990); Medical Research Council (1991).

[111] Mrs Elizabeth Mumford wrote: 'It wasn't really a controversy – just discussion about the meanings of different terms. The US National Commission for the Protection of Human Subjects of Biomedical and Behavioural Research (Belmont Report, 1978) came up with the idea of "minimal risk"; British Paediatric Association (1980) used this interchangeably with "negligible". Then they both tried to define this (e.g. less than that occurring in everyday life). There was subsequent discussion about what these terms really meant and how much risk children faced in everyday life (quite a bit) and whether this was really acceptable, etc. The terms and what they include have changed over time too. For example, the 2004 MRC Ethics Guide (*Medical Research Involving Children*) now describes venepuncture as of "low" rather than "minimal" risk.' E-mails to Ms Caroline Overy, 11 January and 18 February 2012.

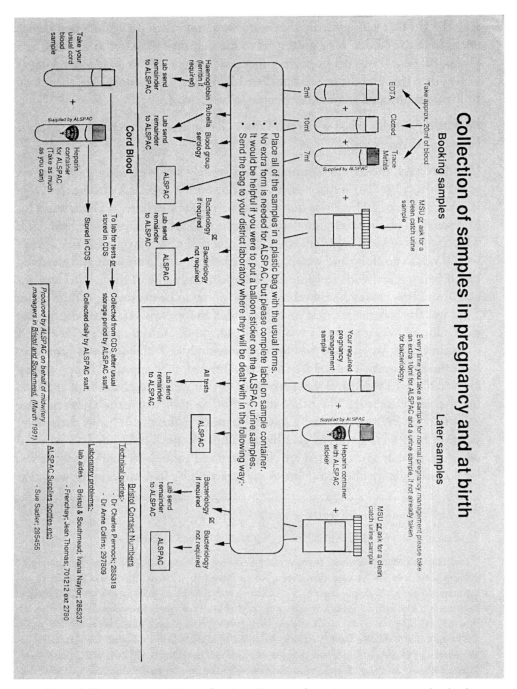

Figure 9: Chart given to midwives for the collection of samples in pregnancy and at birth.

we took seriously from quite an early age. So that's another way in which we resolved the problem.

Peckham: Very interesting. Lessons to be learned for now, I think.

Sadler: If anyone is interested in seeing pictures of a child going through this, I have a set in these documents, so I'll leave those around at the end (see Figure 8). I also have a copy of the chart that we gave to all the midwives to show them what needed to be done at different stages (see Figure 9). That's quite impressive when you think of how much they had to do, so I'll leave those around at the end.

Peckham: There still is a general view that you can't take blood from children, and probably you've got to put this into a context where it can be done easily and safely. Marcus, would you like to tell us when the genetic issues were first discussed?

Pembrey: Yes. I think it's important to go back a bit because the genetics community, before Jean and I met in Athens,[112] had made quite a lot of progress in the 1980s. Some Mendelian disorders had been mapped, there was prenatal diagnosis, carrier testing by linkage, those types of things and, by the end of the 1980s, we started seeing these unusual inheritance patterns. I happen to be involved in this genomic imprinting research,[113] where a gene is only active when transmitted by either the mother or the father. That is, normal DNA was silenced in some way.[114] By that time people were beginning to think that the real challenge was the genetic contributions to the more common disorders, so that was the background.[115] We also have to remember that leading up to 1990 when the Human Genome Project started, with its 15-year projection, there had

---

[112] See page 11.

[113] See Malcolm *et al.* (1991).

[114] Professor Marcus Pembrey wrote: 'To date over 50 genes in the human have been shown to be normally imprinted in a parent-of-origin specific manner, so only a single copy is active. In some the paternal copy is silenced, in the others it is the maternal allele that is silenced. Many imprinted genes are involved in fetal and early growth and development (e.g. insulin growth factor 2), so they are potentially very important in the ALSPAC study. Imprinted genes, discovered in the mid-1980s, are a classic example of epigenetic regulation with gene silencing by DNA methylation rather that DNA sequence change. It is now well established that DNA sequence is complemented by epigenetic information including DNA methylation and histone modifications to determine gene expression.' E-mail to Ms Caroline Overy, 1 January 2012.

[115] For developments in human genetics, see the Wellcome Trust Portfolio Review (2010): 73–80.

been a lot of discussion about whether it would be useful or not.[116] The Human Genome Project was a non-hypothesis-driven study *par excellence.*[117] Quite a bit of that battle for a broad, non-focused approach for the geneticist had already been won, you see, although we were coming from slightly different positions. What happened was that I got involved in discussing the requirements for blood samples and it all hinged on the cell lines. As I've explained, by the summer of 1989 we'd got Porton Down on board, and so it was a question of putting in grant applications for cell lines to the MRC and Wellcome Trust. I can give you a whole list of them,[118] and so on. I was encouraged to put something in but they were never funded. So that opportunity to get cell lines at birth was missed, but we were going to collect blood later as well. The reason why we were emphasizing the cell lines at that time was because I really felt that this might be the only window of opportunity in which to get enough DNA because of the ethical issues. Knowing that the techniques were going to improve over the next 10–15 years, one wanted to be sure that one had enough DNA in order to do all the genetic studies. Imagine if the ethical climate had moved the other way, and we were forbidden from taking blood samples from children other than for their clinical needs. There were all sorts of factors for the reason we wanted to get the cell lines. We failed to get the cell lines for a decade, so we had to then get the consents linked to the samples that had been collected, so we were allowed to do DNA analysis. Before that it was a question of what sort of DNA-banking we should do. So I asked around, you know, 15 000 or 14 000 is a very large number. I seem to remember I went to Bob Williamson at St Mary's[119] because he was somebody you would go and talk to about these things. He said, 'Well, I don't know why you're coming to me. You need to go to Sue Malcolm, the

---

[116] See, for example, Pembrey (1990).

[117] For an introduction to the Human Genome Project, see Fletcher and Porter (1997), and the main Human Genome Project information website at www.ornl.gov/sci/techresources/Human_Genome/home. shtml (visited 1 February 2012).

[118] Professor Marcus Pembrey wrote: 'Two examples of failed grants. 1) Medical Research Council – Pembrey, Marcus; Golding, Jean. "A cell line resource for genetic analysis within the ALSPAC cohort study" 1990 for 5 years; 2) Action Research (S/L2131) – Pembrey, Marcus; Golding, Jean. "A cell line resource for genetic analysis within the Longitudinal Study of Pregnancy and Childhood based on the population of Avon (ALSPAC)" 1991 for 5 years.' E-mail to Ms Caroline Overy, 26 February 2012.

[119] Professor Bob Williamson was professor of molecular genetics at St Mary's Hospital Medical School, Imperial College London (1976–95) after which he moved to the University of Melbourne as director of the Murdoch Institute and professor of medical genetics. He retired in October 2004 and is currently honorary senior principal fellow and professor at the University of Melbourne.

people who are running a clinical service. They may not be doing that number of DNA extractions, but no one else knows anything better about that.' I think it was about 1990/1. I already knew of course that Linda Tyfield was running the clinical molecular and genetic service in Bristol, and that the University of Bristol itself had no academic department of human or medical genetics, rather unusual for a medical school.[120] So I enlisted the help of Linda, to start the ball rolling once we got a grant that allowed us to extract DNA.[121]

Peckham: Did you find it easy to get consent from the parents to look at the DNA?

Pembrey: I was very involved in the wording of the explanation that was given to the mothers about their blood samples, and it said that we would look at their genetics; both theirs and the child, but there was no specifying of which genes. Perhaps we'll come back to that under the ethics section at the end of the afternoon because that's a big story.

Peckham: This was an issue in the Millennium cohort when oral samples were collected. The parents had to be informed that this was not for DNA testing because if it was assumed that samples were used for this purpose parents would not consent.

Pembrey: That was not our experience.

Peckham: You were right in predicting that might have happened.

Pembrey: On the whole, about 70 per cent of the children in the clinics would give a sample for DNA and then at the next clinic, two years later, it would be a different 70 per cent. So in the end we got up to quite large numbers.[122] But to do it chronologically, and go back to the early days; it was a real patchwork. There was a DNA extraction service in Southmead, Bristol, and then the rest of the DNA backing was organized at the Institute of Child Health in London, because there wasn't an equivalent place in Bristol.

---

[120] For the development of clinical genetics as a major medical specialty in Britain, see Harper *et al.* (eds) (2010).

[121] See page 60. Professor Pembrey wrote: 'A two-year grant was gained from the Medical Research Council (£90 000) from 1 February 1995, to J Golding, S Humphries, I Day, M Pembrey, L Tyfield and C Pennock: "Can genetic variation explain Barker's observations concerning fetal growth and adult coronary disease?"' E-mail to Ms Caroline Overy, 1 January 2012.

[122] See Jones *et al.* (2000).

Dr Linda Tyfield: I don't really know what more I can add to that. Perhaps I can say something about the historical context of molecular genetics in Bristol. One point worth making is that we're talking about the early 1990s here, and up until about 1985, in the UK, there were only a few major molecular genetics laboratories that were combining research, a good deal of research, and clinical service work. One was at the Institute of Child Health in London. From about 1985 onwards there was a great burst of local molecular genetics service laboratories serving what were then Regional Health Authorities and some of these were incorporated into existing local pathology service laboratories, such as clinical chemistry or cytogenetics laboratories; others were separate departments.[123] In 1988 I set up a molecular genetics service laboratory in the clinical chemistry department at Southmead Hospital where I had previously been based. There we were in 1991, taking on a very exciting project of extracting DNA from 15 000 samples for ALSPAC when we were still only getting a couple of thousand patient samples a year from the clinical geneticists for specified genetic disorders. We have been concentrating at this meeting today, and quite rightly, on the collection of samples and the inter-relationships between collectors and the mothers and children in the clinics, but one thing that we haven't mentioned yet is the hard work of another group of people – the computing department of ALSPAC. Once the samples were collected, identifying labels were put on those samples, and somehow there had to be a foolproof mechanism to connect a specific sample taken from a specific person at a particular time with all the laboratory data that was eventually going to be generated from that person. If there was an error in the link, the data could be flawed. ALSPAC's computer department had an identifying numbering system which incorporated check digits, rather like our credit cards with the three numbers on the back, that would pick up any transcription errors. The samples were brought to us at Southmead Hospital, from the freezers at United Bristol Healthcare Trust (UBHT) or the Children's Hospital, by various members of the ALSPAC team. The identifying numbers of the samples were originally

---

[123] Dr Tyfield wrote: 'Throughout the 1970s, 1980s and 1990s when there were Regional Health Authorities, monies were top-sliced for specialized laboratory services that were regionally based. Originally these would have included biochemical genetic and cytogenetic services and samples would have come from clinical specialities such as obstetrics and gynaecology, paediatrics, neonatalogy etc. Clinical genetics was another speciality with regional service responsibility and it was in the mid-1980s that molecular genetics laboratories were also included as part of regional specialist services. Originally funding was made available from regional budgets through top-slicing for these regional services. Thereafter the funding process became more complicated.' E-mail to Ms Caroline Overy, 11 December 2011.

entered manually into our ALSPAC-linked computer, and we eventually used a barcode reader. In the beginning there were a number of things we had to test, particularly in relation to the procedures for extracting and aliquoting the DNA. This wasn't as simple as sending a biological sample to a laboratory, putting it into an auto analyser and getting the results out. Not for DNA extraction and genetic analysis at that time, anyway. The gold standard for DNA extraction was the phenol-chloroform method.[124] This was a lengthy, very labour-intensive technique and required several transfers from one tube to another, something that could readily lead to a source of sample mix-up. We had to have checks from a second person at every transfer stage of the process. Although this method was very time-consuming, the reason we stuck with it for so long was that it gave the best quality DNA and the longest lasting high-quality DNA. There were some extraction kits that were commercially available, which yielded perfectly adequate DNA from a fresh blood sample that was suitable for patient analysis in a local service laboratory where only a few genotypes were necessary to provide a clinical result. We needed a technique that ensured a high yield of high-quality, stable DNA, so that years later someone could still go back to these samples and carry out genetic analyses with the assurance that there would be reliable results. The next step was the quality assurance in transferring aliquots of the extracted DNA into multiple-array 96-well polymerase chain reaction (PCR) plates for distribution to our collaborators for genotyping.[125] We included a number of samples in duplicate or triplicate in each 96-well plate in order to ensure the analysis of each plate was done in the correct orientation and that the results were reproducible.[126] Sue Ring may want to say more on this.

---

[124] For the phenol-chloroform method of extracting DNA, see Chomczynski and Sacchi (1987, 2006); Puissant and Houdebine (1990).

[125] Dr Linda Tyfield wrote: 'Collaborators were individuals in research laboratories who were exploring the possible relationship between certain genotypes and particular phenotypes, e.g. the association between variation at an individual locus and the susceptibility to, or potential for, developing a particular condition.' E-mail to Ms Caroline Overy, 15 February 2012.

[126] Dr Linda Tyfield wrote: 'Some of the blood samples that were brought to us had been stored (frozen) for some time and it is almost certain that there would have been some degradation of the DNA during the initial period of storage. The phenol-chloroform method enables extraction of long, intact DNA as well as shorter, degraded strands. At the time we started extracting the DNA, PCR (the polymerase chain reaction) was in use everywhere. This is an ingenious technique whereby millions of copies of a particular part of the genome could be made in a tiny tube thereby making it possible to examine/analyse the DNA sequence in that specific area. A great advantage of PCR is that really top quality DNA is not always needed (although it certainly is an advantage) at the beginning of the reaction because the aim is to amplify a specific area of the genome.' E-mail to Ms Caroline Overy, 20 December 2012.

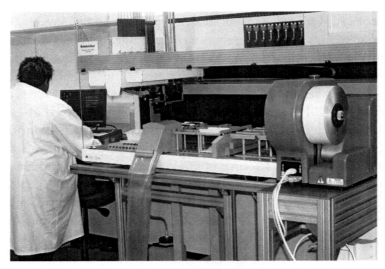

Figure 10. Robobanker robot. In 2003, ALSPAC acquired two robots to immortalize cell lines. They were named by cohort members, the 'Germinator' which grew cells and 'Robobanker' (pictured) which stored them.

Ring: I was first employed as a post-doc on the first major DNA-banking grant at the end of 1996 in Linda Tyfield's lab. I'd come from a genetics research background and I think one of the most important things that happened in the development of the DNA bank was that it was set up in a clinical service laboratory. I learned an awful lot from working in Linda's lab, and also with Richard Jones, regarding the quality control steps that we needed to put in place to have a DNA bank that can still be used this far in the future. I think that was one of the crucial things; it wasn't just seen as a finite research project, it had the long-term forethought to use the appropriate quality control procedures. As Linda said, we had to try several different methods to try to work out which DNA extraction method was best to use. One thing that Linda didn't say in her summary was that one of the problems was that, by the time I was employed, the samples were already seven to eight years old. The commercial kits available at the time were good if you had samples that were relatively recent. I'd test kits out on test blood that was two months old, and then move over to the precious ALSPAC samples, and it just wouldn't work because they'd been in storage for too long. In fact, in the laboratory, we're still using phenol-chloroform extraction if we're extracting samples that have been in the freezers for a long time. We had tracking systems in the lab, we started using barcodes from the seven-year clinic.[127] Regarding the strategy for setting up the bank: we started

---

[127] See pages 60–1.

by extracting DNA from cord blood, but that blood was collected in heparin anticoagulant and, at the time, this was problematic as heparin inhibited PCR in the genotyping processes. That's not an issue any more,[128] but back then it was, and so we had to rethink the whole strategy of which samples to use first. Therefore when I first started we were going to create the children's DNA bank first, but then we had to put that on hold and move to the mothers' samples, which were collected in ethylenediaminetetraacetic acid (EDTA),[129] and wait until the seven-year clinic to start the children's collection. So there was quite a lot of rejigging of plans due to the state of the samples at the time. When the samples left our laboratory they were taken to Richard in London to process, and at this point I'll hand over to Richard.

Jones: One of the interesting things at an early stage was trying to assess how the identity of individual samples would be preserved. I think it would be true to say that we discovered that people are very bad beyond numbers in the tens or hundreds, in keeping track of what they've done to a particular sample. The beauty of moving to a robotic system is that, unlike a person, a robot does what you tell it to do and it does it exactly, even if you've got it wrong.

What we were doing was taking an industrial pharmaceutical way of dealing with large numbers of samples and learning how to work these systems and put them in a research context. I think the interesting thing was how the idea of using robotics in a university study seemed to be quite foreign to people, whereas, in fact, if you looked at what was happening in industry, this was commonplace and being used extensively. It was at that point also that we started to widely use barcodes that prevented samples from being muddled up. There's nothing much more to say about that really except that it was good fun. [Laughter]

Peckham: When was the DNA available for researchers? How long did this process take?

Pembrey: Well, I think we ought to backtrack a little bit here: obviously there was the question of extracting the DNA, but the whole question of banking it was something that we had to address before we could put in the big strategic grant to the Medical Research Council. This was for £1 million in order to employ

---

[128] Dr Sue Ring wrote: 'Methods have been developed which use less DNA therefore the effects of heparin can be overcome by diluting the samples.' E-mail to Ms Caroline Overy, 30 January 2012.

[129] Dr Sue Ring wrote: 'Ethylenediaminetetraacetic acid (EDTA) is an anticoagulant used as heparin is used to prevent blood clotting.' E-mail to Ms Caroline Overy, 30 January 2012.

people like Sue Ring and others, and actually fund the robots.[130] I asked around, and there wasn't much expertise on this that I could find at the Institute of Child Health, and I was quite concerned about it. Then it happened that the job in clinical pathology was vacant at the Institute and Great Ormond Street. Doug Higgs, who is somebody who worked with David Weatherall[131] told me that Richard Jones was in the market, as it were, and indeed he was appointed. What particularly interested me about this episode was David Weatherall, who had written a letter to me right at the beginning when I approached him in 1988/9, saying what a wonderful idea ALSPAC was and so forth and so on, although we had singularly failed to get any money for the genetic aspects and the DNA bank at all. In 1992, I think it was, I had to go up to Oxford on a site visit: they were on the receiving end and I was chairing the site visit.[132] I said to David: 'Oh, could I have a word before we get started at 9 o'clock?' And he said, 'Yes, come into my office,' and before I could say: 'What do you think of Richard Jones because we're thinking of approaching him to come to the Institute?' he said, 'I know what you're going to talk about, you're going to talk about ALSPAC' and was trying to explain why we hadn't got any funding.[133] So anyway, Richard came to work with us and it was a long old haul to get the robots to work.

Jones: The problem was not primarily getting the robots to work, the problem was finding out how much DNA we had in each sample, and how much we were giving away. The reason for that is that people had believed that they were measuring the concentration of DNA samples in the past, and in fact they weren't, because DNA is so difficult to deal with. Those of you who have dealt with it know that it's gloopy, and moving accurate quantities of gloopy material around is almost impossible. We were being pressured by potential collaborators, who said: 'What's the delay? This is a very simple business.' They didn't know

---

[130] Professor Marcus Pembrey wrote: 'A four-year grant from the Medical Research Council (£1 009 207) from 19 May 1997 to M Pembrey, J Golding, H Simmons, L Tyfield, R Jones for development of a DNA resource for genetic studies within ALSPAC.' E-mail to Ms Caroline Overy, 1 January 2012.

[131] Professor Douglas Higgs is currently professor of molecular haematology at the University of Oxford and director of the MRC Molecular Haematology Unit; Professor Sir David Weatherall was Regius Professor of Medicine (1992–2000) and is retired honorary director of the Weatherall Institute of Molecular Medicine at the University of Oxford.

[132] Professor Marcus Pembrey wrote: 'This was a site visit for renewal of an Action Research grant to David Weatherall'. E-mail to Ms Caroline Overy, 1 January 2012.

[133] From the Wellcome Trust; Professor Sir David Weatherall was a governor of the Wellcome Trust from 1990–2000.

that it was not a simple business. We knew that it was not a simple business, and it took us some time to get to the point where we had confidence when people asked us for a sample of DNA, that we could give them a certain quantity. The problem is now well recognized, but has been quite chronic. I have to confess, though, looking back on it, that I sometimes wonder that, given the difficulties of measuring DNA concentration and attempting to aliquot it out in constant amounts for collaborators, whether in fact had we simply put a drop in the bottom of a tube, not knowing how much was there, and distributed that, I'd be interested to know what the comparison was and the quality of genetic results from the totally untouched set of samples, compared with those to which we'd tried our utmost to get the concentrations even and equal. I don't know the answer to that, but sometimes you have to ask these questions.

Pembrey: We're getting to answer your question as to when the DNA was available. What happened was that we had one project grant from the MRC in 1994/5, in which we were going to start doing DNA extractions in Linda's lab. But in order to get the strategic funding for DNA-banking from the MRC, we obviously needed a national advisory committee. So in 1995 we formed a genetics advisory committee, and I was chairing it. Linda, of course, was on it; there was John Todd; Alex Markham, who was going to be here today; Ian Day, a technical adviser; Jean Golding; Steve Humphries from UCL; and Richard Jones; and David Baum attended some of the early meetings.[134] At the first meeting of that group, one thing we had to consider was applications for studying a particular gene; we didn't want, in those days, a lot of duplication of genetic analysis. Both John Todd and Steve Humphries wanted to study the insulin growth factor 2, and so the first time we had a fight on. There was only one gene they wanted to study and it was the same one. [Laughter] But we persuaded them to sort it out between themselves. In those days we would only be studying the 'Children in Focus' samples, and we would receive applications for the genes that people wanted to study and then discuss them gene by gene in this committee, which met several times a year. The first paper eventually got published in 1998, so it was

---

[134] Professor John Todd was then senior scientist, at the Wellcome Trust Centre for Human Genetics, Nuffield Department of Surgery, University of Oxford (now professor of medical genetics, Cambridge University); Professor Sir Alex Markham has been professor of medicine, Leeds Institute of Molecular Medicine, since 1992; Professor Ian Day held a British Heart Foundation Intermediate Fellowship at UCL Medical School (now professor of molecular and genetic epidemiology, Bristol Genetic Epidemiology Laboratories); Professor Steve Humphries was at the Centre for Genetics of Cardiovascular Disorders at UCL Medical School (now British Heart Foundation professor of cardiovascular genetics at UCL).

a long time from when the DNA was originally taken.[135] Today, of course, the idea of discussing gene by gene what you were analysing would be complete nonsense.

Peckham: What did you charge them for the samples?

Pembrey: This is a very good point because we didn't have full funding at this time, we hadn't got to the stage of any core funding from the Wellcome Trust, for example, so we had to try and claw back some money. It was quite a large amount; I can't remember – Sue Ring, do you remember? A lot of people were put off from doing the study because they would get a thousand DNAs but it would cost them, you know, £11 000 or £12 000, something like that.[136]

Jones: I was going to comment more given that Marcus has gone into the business of dealing with collaborators. It is interesting to look back to that point where each individual collaborator would have one or a few genes in mind, and was particularly keen that they should have a sample of DNA in their hands. So their view of the resource was as a source of actual, physical DNA and that participating as a collaborator was to actually go away with that DNA. I think then, over time, the idea that there would be a pool of genetic information, independent of the actual samples, which was itself a paper resource, slowly took over; potential collaborators became far more relaxed about whether they were doing the actual DNA analysis or whether someone else was going to do it, and they would be given the information. That has probably moved on steadily now, and I think George Davey Smith, from what you were telling me today, we have now reached the point where DNA is not being handed out particularly to individuals because you're collecting the information across the whole genome.

Davey Smith: Yes, most of the requests now are for genetic data rather than for samples of the DNA because we have genome-wide data; 600 000+ markers on virtually everyone on whom we have samples.[137] Thus the requests for DNA are fewer. There are requests for samples for methylation (epigenetic) analysis,[138] of course, which I guess wasn't something considered earlier on. Marcus could

---

[135] Dunger *et al.* (1998).

[136] Professor Marcus Pembrey wrote: 'The figures for "claw back" on DNA-banking costs from non-Wellcome Trust or MRC-funded projects ended up in 2003 as £10 000 for 1000 DNAs and £40 000 for 10 000 DNAs.' Note on draft transcript, 26 September 2011.

[137] For example, the ALSPAC genome-wide data is included in Paternoster *et al.* (2010).

[138] For further information on epigenetics see Relton and Davey Smith (2010).

say whether this would have been a possibility all those years ago. For us today, bioinformatics and data handling issues are key.

Peckham: I think the whole issue of the data linkage, or the linkage of genetic information to the general ALSPAC database is interesting. Are you talking about analysis of the samples with linkage to the information in ALSPAC, or just analysis of the samples when people are requesting samples from specific groups within the cohort?

Jones: It's retrieving the genetic data from the actual DNA samples. That's what I'm calling analysis.

Peckham: Yes, but they wanted that without any information from the ALSPAC cohort? Because that's another issue, isn't it?

Jones: Yes. There are perhaps some questions you can ask about that.

Golding: We had a very complex system whereby every set of data, whether it was a questionnaire or a biological sample of the DNA, had its own number, and the number had check digits at the end, so that if you mistyped it, it would show as an error. Then there was a complex set of programmes that would link these things together. You wouldn't be able to do it if you came across one data set and another yourself, so that applied to the DNA in just the same way as anything else; at least that's my understanding of how it worked. But that was thanks to our computer team, which worked all the hours God gave them.

Jones: The interesting development was from individual collaborators very much wanting their own bit of DNA from which they could extract the genetic data themselves, and so on, over a course of, what are we talking about, ten years? In ten years we've arrived at a situation where it's essentially an industrial process, generating data efficiently for everybody, and not bit by bit. The important thing is to contrast that achievement with the other part, the blood samples, the plasma, or the serum or whatever you've stored, where there had always been promise of a similar kind of development, but as far as I know, this has hardly happened; which means that there is an enormous stress on biological sample collection outside DNA, in the sense that it's still accessed by individuals who don't necessarily have the most efficient way of extracting their biochemical or biological data from the sample. Those samples are finite; you can't amplify them as you can DNA, and they are constantly being used in a relatively inefficient way. It's very hard to resist the inefficient use because each inefficient use is linked to a grant and each grant is bringing money to the study. There has been no real rational development in the same way as there has with genetics in the whole field of other biological data.

Pembrey: Could I just add two points? The first is to illustrate the hand-to-mouth way in which we worked. When we were able to get the £1 million DNA-banking grant at the end of 1995/beginning of 1996, a large bit of the money was for the computing backup, actually for the DNA database and so forth. But the situation was that we were getting the DNA at the seven-year clinic and there wasn't any money for the computing needed for the appointments for the seven-year old clinic. So quite a bit of the DNA money was used for that purpose. Quite rightly, because the idea was to get DNA at the end of it.

Another point is that at a fairly early advisory committee of one sort or another, I remember George Davey Smith saying that we have to get 3 per cent duplicates; that with people coming through the clinic we have to get 3 per cent who would go through it all again. The issue was whether they would give blood samples again? George said, 'Yes, of course, otherwise you can't know A, B, and C.'[139] I remember this being discussed in the Law and Ethics Committee, whether to take a second blood sample or not. In fact, it has proved absolutely vital, very useful, particularly in the early days, for validating whether labs were able to do genetic analysis. We had this check – they wouldn't know, of course, which were the duplicates.[140] So those two points helped launch and maintain the standard of the DNA-bank.

Davey Smith: I was going to say something else, but I remember having to go to the Ethics Committee to present this, as being a very scary occasion, but we constantly have to report the coefficients of variation for such measures in papers, so it has been useful.[141] One further point, which doesn't really relate to the history, but on Richard's point: there is this promise of proteomics, metabonomics, measuring everything in a tiny blood sample.[142] The technology is still developing.

---

[139] Professor Marcus Pembrey wrote: 'The 3 per cent figure was arbitrary, it was just that we needed a reasonable number of repeat analyses on the same subject to judge the reproducibility of the methods and procedures used.' E-mail to Ms Caroline Overy, 26 February 2012. See note 141.

[140] For an example of validating a laboratory with duplicate samples for kidney dialysis, see comments made by Dr Felix Konotey-Ahulu in Crowther *et al.* (eds) (2009): 41–2.

[141] For a report of these coefficients of variation see, for example, Donald *et al.* (2010).

[142] Professor George Davey Smith wrote: 'Proteomics and metabonomics are methods that measure a very large number of factors in small samples of blood or urine. For this approach see, for example, Chadeau-Hyam *et al.* (2011).' E-mail to Ms Caroline Overy, 9 December 2011.

The problem with those technologies at the moment is that they don't give people what they want because they essentially give you the size of particles in the blood, but they don't tell you how much there is of this particular analyte or that analyte. But when we're down to limited samples, we certainly have a policy of not allowing those to be used for a single or a couple of analytes, but saving samples in the belief that eventually the technology will develop to the level where they can produce the type of useful information on very large numbers of particular analytes.

Jones: I think the DNA example, the genetics example, is just an example of how it was at the beginning, although you had to wait a long time for a grant application to work; when there was money, the money was very generous by comparison with any other part of ALSPAC. I was a beneficiary of that. It goes to show that the amount of effort and fragmentary financing of a study creates enormous problems and inefficiencies. When you suddenly get, what was it, £2 million or something, when you magically get funded on an adequate level to do something, the gains in efficiency are so large. I think the only block is the fear of a white elephant, isn't it? There's an enormous cost to that and I think ALSPAC has always managed to get through that in piecemeal fashion, but at many stages it would have been so much more efficient if someone had had the courage of their conviction, in giving us that £2 million, when the children were aged five or six.

Peckham: It's extraordinary really that the momentum was kept up for so long until you were able to reach that stage.

Jones: Indeed. Well, that's down to Jean, I think.

Golding: Down to everybody.

Peckham: Can I ask you, Jean, about the broader issue of collaboration because data access and collaboration is very important? I am aware of recent changes, but if researchers want access to your data, how did you deal with that? Was it a big issue for you? I know it was perceived as an issue by some outside, and it must have been difficult for you given your resources and support.

Golding: The issue was over finances, and people who had worked with the big national cohort studies were used to getting data free from those studies,[143] which

---

[143] Most cohort data can be accessed by registering with the UK Data Archive, which is administered by the Economic and Social Data Service (ESDS) at the University of Essex, www.esds.ac.uk/longitudinal/ (visited 16 November 2011). ESDS Longitudinal has undertaken a data audit of ALSPAC in preparation for improved access for secondary users and, from June 2009, a set of sampler data files produced by the ALSPAC study team was available at www.esds.ac.uk/findingdata/snDescription.asp?sn=6147 (visited 16 November 2011).

was natural because the data had been paid for and archived so that they could be obtained. We asked for collaborators to raise some money towards our costs of collecting the data, and a number of people found that a big issue. We were, we thought, always being very collaborative and always looked at proposals; it was the steering committee or the scientific advisory committee that considered them all, and made suggestions or, very rarely, turned any down. One of the things one had to look at was the ethics as well as the science.

Peckham: Did the research councils accept that? If people put in an application to do a study, did they accept the fact that payment was included in the proposal?

Golding: They did eventually. It took the ESRC until the 2000s to do so. The MRC accepted it much earlier. The Wellcome Trust finally accepted it.[144] But we were asking for about £40 000 per grant, which for running the study was great because it wasn't tied to any particular thing, so you could plug a hole or two with it.

Peckham: So now with more adequate funding, has access to data and collaboration been made easier? Is that right, George?

Davey Smith: Yes, and it also became a condition of funding on a proper basis, if you like. As you are very well aware, in this building of the Wellcome Trust (215 Euston Road), they particularly drove the line that when they were funding studies like ALSPAC they were funded as resources rather than as single studies based in single places. That is now a condition of the funding. But there are still extensive amounts of funding raised through collaborative activities, in particular activities that fund additional aspects of data collection, so that the core funding support funds a skeleton operation collecting rather minimal levels of data, and certainly from the last 15+ and 17+ clinics, more of the funding has been the additional funding than has actually been the core support. That funding has to be built in in advance to support the actual collection of the data; we are not going ahead to collect the data and then obtain funding for its use. I think if I ran up an overdraft of £1 million at Bristol University today, I would come in to find my desk emptied and be escorted off the premises.

Peckham: I'm sure you would. Would anyone like to say any more on the genetic aspects? We've got a few more minutes, and I would like to go back to the issue of governance because I think this has been a terribly important aspect, an aspect

---

[144] Professor Jean Golding wrote: 'As far as we can tell, the Wellcome Trust started allowing a fee for ALSPAC in 1998, and the MRC in 2000.' E-mail to Ms Caroline Overy, 20 December 2011.

that has, as you mentioned, informed Biobank and a lot of the other studies; it's been a real example. Can we go back and discuss it a bit more fully? Also the changes in ethics committees and how they function. You've seen those changes while trying to retain control of the study. I think the tension is quite interesting.

Mumford: I've been associated with the Ethics Committee for 21 years; I was there at its first meeting, but I'm still convinced that the most important period in the life of that committee was the gestational period, that is the period before we all arrived. In my view it's quite remarkable that the committee came to exist at all, particularly with the very broad mandate that it had. To understand that you have to go back, as you say, to look at the state of the ethical regulation, of the legal regulation, of medical research 20 or 25 years ago. I dug out a couple of old textbooks of medical law. Let me read one to you: this one was by Mason and McCall Smith, who has, of course, become better known for other sorts of writing, but he is a wonderful writer of medical law as well. This is a quotation from the second edition (1989):[145]

> It is now almost mandatory for hospitals or health authorities to establish 'ethical committees' whose function is to sanction each experimental project before it is launched. Despite the fact that the setting up of committees was advised as long ago as 1967, their composition and remit is still not firmly based. Their existence is, however, becoming more widespread.[146]

The book goes on to question whether there ought to be lay members on such committees. In another paper written around the same time the author had done a survey of ethics committees, and reported that the membership ranged from anything between 3 to 15 members, and the meetings from anything between never to once a month.[147] I know that ethical scrutiny in one university with which I was associated, was done by having proposed projects sent from the

---

[145] Mason and McCall Smith (1989): 256. Alexander McCall Smith is now more widely known as a writer of fiction, for example, *The No. 1 Ladies Detective Agency* series.

[146] Following the World Medical Association's Declaration of Helsinki (ethical principles for medical research involving human subjects) in 1964 (see Riis (2001)) and the publication of Pappworth's *Human Guinea Pigs* (1967), the Royal College of Physicians recommended that all research be subject to ethical review (Royal College of Physicians (1967)). See also Reynolds and Tansey (2007).

[147] See Nicholson (ed.) (1986).

medical school to the law school; the law professors then, as part of their *pro bono* work, simply went through the papers, gave an answer, and sent everything back to the medical school. So ethical scrutiny was haphazard, and, if you look at the 'law professors versus medical professors' example, it was a bit adversarial.[148]

Of course, the whole area of the regulation of medical research grew out of the experiences, the atrocities of Nazi Germany, the Nuremberg trials and the Nuremberg Code.[149] It's a bit of an unfortunate way to start, but I think that relationship did mark, and probably still does mark to some extent, the relationship between ethics committees and people trying to do medical research. At the same time, 20 years ago, possibly even more than now, there was a real fear, I think, among the scientific and medical community about what they called 'defensive medicine'. There were a lot of articles being written about the threat coming from the US of this imposition on clinical practice, and also on medical research.[150] So you got the haphazard, the adversarial, and then along comes ALSPAC. There was a lot of writing done at the time, in the 1980s, about good ethical practice. We've talked about the guidelines from the British Paediatric Association (Royal College of Paediatrics and Child Health since 1996), the Royal College of Physicians and so forth.[151] I still think it's groundbreaking that the founders of ALSPAC had this idea, not of submitting reluctantly to scrutiny, but actually asking for help and collaboration. That's really the outstanding thing about the beginning of this committee: the sense that having an ethically ideal study was every bit as important as having a scientifically ideal study.

---

[148] Mrs Elizabeth Mumford wrote: 'It is the idea of scientists having no participation in the ethical scrutiny and the slight rivalry between law and medical faculties – it's always easier to grumble about the results when it's "them vs us".' E-mail to Ms Caroline Overy, 11 January 2012.

[149] 'The Nuremberg Code was the first internationally recognized set of guidelines dealing specifically with non-therapeutic human experimentation.' Hazelgrove (2001): 559.

[150] Mrs Elizabeth Mumford wrote: 'It's hard to know the extent to which this ever really did or does happen in the UK. Certainly there have been dozens of articles about it in the US – mostly about its financial cost. The fear of it spreading was certainly widespread, probably more so in the 1980s than now. The term is intended to refer to unnecessary tests and procedures done in order to protect clinicians against potential legal action. Clinical judgement might suggest that there was no need for the procedure, but nothing is ever certain in medicine and so the fear that the unlikely might materialize, and the untested/untreated patient complain and sue, might lead to something being done "just in case". Such procedures may, of course, also be detrimental to the patient, if they themselves carry risks. As for particular examples, caesarean section is one commonly cited, as are CT scans for every head injury. But are these really examples of defensive medicine, or just an example of our risk-averse culture?' E-mail to Ms Caroline Overy, 18 February 2012.

[151] See note 110.

My own involvement with ALSPAC began when I got a letter from Professor Michael Furmston[152] in the Bristol law faculty inviting me to come along and join the Ethics Committee. I was very excited; it was my first year as a lecturer, and this was a thrilling opportunity for me. I think the enthusiasm for that committee is the same sort of enthusiasm that marked the whole of the ALSPAC study. The fact that this committee was not just to be a reactive one, but a proactive one, something that other people have mentioned already, made it particularly interesting to be in at the beginning. I also think that some of the most interesting work done by the committee was done in the first year. As for the issues, if you look at the minutes of the first year, all the issues were there.[153]

Michael Furmston began the first meeting by saying: 'Now these are the things we've got to look at.' He began with consent: consent to take part at all; consent to answer questions; consent to make use of biological samples. A year and a half on, that was the first issue that the committee had disagreements about.[154] It was the first time that we couldn't actually reach a conclusion on the spot. We came back again and again to look at biological samples, and finally decided how we were going to get consent for them – the way in which that was going to be handled. So we looked at consent in that first meeting.

We also looked at confidentiality and talked about the postal questionnaires, and the interviews. It might have been at that meeting that we first came across a phrase which has come back again and again to haunt us; the statement that there was no way that participants' names and the information they provided

---

[152] See note 71.

[153] Mrs Elizabeth Mumford wrote: 'In the minutes of the very first meeting, we outlined the issues of: 1. Consent (a) to join the study/fill in questionnaires/be interviewed and (b) to physical tests (e.g. blood, placenta); 2. Confidentiality; 3. Access to information – i.e. reporting of results and 4. Use of biological samples'. E-mail to Ms Caroline Overy, 11 January 2012.

[154] Mrs Elizabeth Mumford wrote: 'The problem was essentially that the best time for taking samples (i.e. when they were being obtained for therapeutic reasons in any case) was not necessarily the best time for obtaining consent to ALSPAC's research. The consent might well be obtained months later. Samples taken early on would be of no use after a lengthy storage period, and it was much more efficient and led to better scientific research etc to batch them and do some preliminary work on them as soon as they became available. However, ALSPAC participants had been told at the outset that research would not be undertaken on their samples until they had given consent. The divergent points of view were as follows: some believed that there was no real problem as: (1) ALSPAC was just generating raw data, not really doing research yet; (2) what people were really worried about was confidentiality and that would certainly be respected; (3) it wasn't even strictly necessary to obtain consent to use the leftover bits of tissue already taken for therapeutic purposes. On the other hand, others felt essentially that a promise was a promise – whatever the form of words.' E-mails to Ms Caroline Overy, 11 January and 18 February 2012.

could be linked. Right from the beginning we also considered the question of access to information; whether we were going to report things back to the participants. Gordon has already talked about some of the problems we've had and some of the conclusions that we reached as to how much information to give back.[155] But all of this came up in the first meeting.

The work of the committee has been not only interesting, it's also been very enjoyable. In its early days I think that this was in large measure because of the personality of its first chairman, Michael Furmston. His style of easygoing, congenial leadership has, I think, been taken over by Gordon and David Jewell,[156] who have subsequently been the chairmen. Michael Furmston is now the dean of a law faculty in Singapore; he retired from Bristol 12 or 13 years ago. If you haven't met him, he is a man who is 'larger than life' in every way. He was twice dean of the Bristol law faculty, he was Pro Vice-Chancellor, an eminent scholar in contract and commercial law, areas of law miles away from this one. He is a barrister, a practising barrister. He would lead the meetings in a style, which I suppose is reminiscent of the development of the common law, so he'd do it by stories and anecdotes. Some of them were anecdotes about his own home life – quite a lot of them were – but his home life was rather interesting as well. He had ten children, plus about 22 dogs, and goats, and I believe some other type of small animal. They bred animals to show. He was a postal chess champion. He was an expert on the American Civil War and on cricket. To find him in his office you would first have to negotiate a sort of labyrinth of bookshelves. But he was enthusiastic, he was warm, he was encouraging, and he had a wonderful style of leading meetings. So it made it a very civilized, very enjoyable atmosphere in which to conduct some really very difficult business. I think that's what made the committee such a success in its early days. Many people have remarked since then that this pattern of real collaboration has continued: collaboration amongst the members of the committee and with the study. We felt that we were working on this together to get answers that would be beneficial to the study as a whole.

Peckham: So it was much more than an ethics committee?

Mumford: Far more than that. We looked at individual projects as they came along, but we were looking far more to the future, thinking how we would

---

[155] See page 35.

[156] Dr David Jewell is the current chair of the ALSPAC Law and Ethics Committee; he was a senior lecturer in primary health care in the University of Bristol from 1987 to 1999.

handle these issues and discussing things in that sort of broad sense. I think that's what makes it quite different, and probably remains in some ways different, from almost any other ethics committee, although there are some which have followed in its wake. In the early days, I presented a couple of papers on the work of the Committee and people from other European countries would come up and say: 'This is really exciting. Nobody else does this.' That distinction was the idea of the people who came up with the proposal for the committee in the first place.[157]

Peckham: So what is the situation now with the current ALSPAC, George, in terms of your relationship with the Ethics Committee given the other developments which have taken place around ethics more widely? Does it still have the same role, or has it changed?

Davey Smith: No, I think it has exactly the same role and David Jewell is the current chairperson. Obviously there has always been a sort of dual structure, in that there are what are now called the National Research Ethics Service (NRES) committees, and studies that involved NHS facilities or any invasive procedures such as taking blood or scans, etc., go to the NRES. There's also the faculty ethics committee in the university, which the ALSPAC Ethics Committee works with, and we have discussions with people who are in different faculties who go through their ethics committees. So there's a complex web of ethics committees, which, I think, reflects the fact that there is basically no single legal foundation for the role and function of these committees. The ALSPAC Ethics Committee certainly has had an absolutely vital role in the study.

Peckham: Have you had any disagreements with the national ethics committees in some of your decisions?

Davey Smith: I think disagreements would be the wrong term. Many things have been iterative. Marcus alluded to this earlier and, though it didn't really come up in the discussion here about genetics, this was a big area. There were definitely big changes in perspectives regarding the ethical issues and around genetic analysis, when the earlier notions were that we got marker-by-marker approval, which has become unfeasible. Although it wasn't in ALSPAC but in another study I was involved in running, our approach was to send frequent applications to the committee until this was realized as not to be sustainable. Then bodies such as the MRC started developing statements regarding appropriate ethical approvals

---

[157] Mumford (1999a and b).

with respect to genetic analysis.[158] There was also a change in the gestalt around what genetic analysis was going to tell you as it started becoming clear that, with common genetic variants, the effect sizes were going to be small and were not going to have individual level implications. I think it would be wrong to put that under the heading as a 'disagreement', but it went through iterations where it went through the ALSPAC Law and Ethics Committee, back to our local LREC as it was then, and I was asked to attend them during that period, and decisions emerged. It didn't appear to be a conflictive situation, but was a situation where the procedures needed to change, if you like, to fit both the technology and what had become known.

Peckham: The continuity in the discussions we've had has been very interesting – how the study has grown and developed.

Mumford: I think in the early days we were considered quite tough. I think our standards were a little bit more stringent, and some researchers would say: 'Look, the LREC has approved this project. What's wrong with you? Why are you so much more stringent in what you're requiring?' Looking over the early minutes that sort of response came up a few times.[159]

Golding: I want to put on record that I found the Ethics Committee somewhat scary, but incredibly helpful. In retrospect, yes. But I could approach them with problems I'd had or a decision that I'd had to make quickly, and then we could discuss it afterwards and record what had happened and what should happen in the future. I found the whole thing was a positive support, in what were very hairy situations at times because things were moving so fast.

Mumford: And you'd be there and we'd ask you: 'Please Jean, can you explain to us what this is all about?' There really was a sense of collaboration.

Stirrat: Perhaps there's one small area that hasn't been picked up, which is an important one, and related to the interviewers who would be going out to homes.

---

[158] For the MRC ethics and research guidance, see www.mrc.ac.uk/Ourresearch/Ethicsresearch guidance/index.htm (visited 20 December 2011); for the Wellcome Trust guidelines on ethical practice, see www.wellcome.ac.uk/About-us/Policy/Policy-and-position-statements/WTD002753.htm (visited 20 December 2011).

[159] Mrs Elizabeth Mumford wrote: 'I have one set of minutes that refers to Dr X (a collaborator who was a frequent visitor to the committee) who highlighted the difference between the local research ethics committee's response to his proposed research (permission to test "spare" biological material without the consent of the mother) and ALSPAC's response (no testing without the prior consent of the mother).' E-mail to Ms Caroline Overy, 11 January 2012.

On occasions they came across situations that distressed them, and indeed really needed to be reported: potential child abuse, these sorts of things. One of the things that we did early on in the Committee was to set down the criteria and the mechanisms through which it was ethical, legal and appropriate to bring those situations to the attention of the appropriate authorities. It was actually Jean, I think, and she might want to comment on that. That was important not only for the whole conduct of the committee and of ALSPAC, but for those interviewers themselves because it gave them backup. They actually felt they were supported.

Golding: Yes, things were reported to me first and then I reported them to Alan who was the community paediatrician.

Emond: One of the most difficult things in my involvement with ALSPAC was trying to balance my responsibilities as a clinician participating in safeguarding children in the NHS with my responsibilities to the study. I felt that ALSPAC had to adopt the same thresholds of concern as were current in clinical practice. There were a couple of occasions where it did result in the family withdrawing from the study, and that caused a lot of heartache, but I think my conscience is clear that, at the end of the day, we did pertain to the same thresholds that were around at the time. Again, over time, these thresholds have changed, and probably have got lower rather than higher, but ALSPAC did take these seriously. There were one or two quite worrying cases of neglect and abuse, and of mental health issues, that we had to take account of. These are not written up anywhere, but that did go on behind the scenes. I'm sure Jean had some troubled nights about these cases, because you were caught in a dilemma, because you knew if you blew the whistle the family would withdraw from the study, and on a couple of occasions we had to do that.

Golding: I should point out that this only occurred where it was direct contact with the participants. Anything written in the questionnaires was not acted upon. That was always something that one could talk about with the Ethics Committee.

Peckham: Are there any other burning questions you think that we haven't covered that you'd like to mention?

Birmingham: I took over from Elizabeth Mumford as secretary of the Ethics Committee. There's just one thing that seems to me to be a bit of a problem with all ethics committees, whether it's our own or the LREC as well, and that is consistency. It seems that it's very difficult for them to be consistent. David Jewell, our current chair with the ALSPAC Ethics Committee, talks about that now and it seems that we need to have some policies that are made and approved by the Ethics Committee, so it's quite clear. There are a lot of areas where there isn't a policy written for it, and it will come up two years, three years, four years later. I regard part of my job to look back and see what the committee decided and when this was talked about earlier? Things change: the gestalt of ethics changes.

Peckham: Can you given an example?

Birmingham: Of inconsistency?

Peckham: Yes, of something that might have cropped up.

Birmingham: Well, I can certainly give you a very good example of inconsistency from the LREC, where we put in an application to take blood from parents who accompanied the children to the clinic. Because we ran annual clinics, and we're a 21-month cohort, there were two clinics running at the same time. So one application went in as part of a new application for this particular clinic, that we'd like to take the blood from the parents, along with all the other measures. The other was an amendment to a clinic already running. It was exactly the same paperwork, apart from the heading: Team Focus 1 or Team Focus 2, or whatever – they went to the same committee on the same day. One was approved with no comment; the other was not approved with a great long list of reasons why we couldn't use blood from those parents without further ethical approval for each proposed analysis. That caused us huge difficulties. Three years later, George eventually managed to sort it out. We had this one set of blood that was collected at this particular clinic which we couldn't use. You couldn't just go back to them and say: 'Well, hang on a minute. You've approved it here, but not here.' It took three years to sort out.[160] It was really frustrating.

---

[160] Miss Karen Birmingham wrote: 'Just to clarify, blood collection (with informed broad consent for future research) from parents accompanying their children to the ALSPAC research clinic for 12-year olds, was approved without comment. For parents accompanying their children to the very similar research clinic for 13-year olds, using identical consent forms, the LREC stipulated that "... any proposed research involving this collection of DNA and cell lines thereof should be subject to further ethical review by the Research Ethics Committee as per MRC guideline. Approval in terms of this application is only for the collection and storage of these samples." This was not only a misinterpretation of the MRC guidelines, but also totally inconsistent between the two clinics. The blood was taken and stored and not wasted, but it took a very long time before they agreed to us using the cell lines and DNA without gaining further consent.' E-mail to Ms Caroline Overy, 9 December 2011.

Peckham: Are there any other relevant topics that you feel are important? It's been fascinating listening to the historical development of ALSPAC.

Tansey: It really has. I'd like to thank you all very much for coming and telling us your stories, and actually shedding so much light on an important study. I'm very grateful to you all for coming and contributing. As I said at the beginning, we will be in touch with you throughout the rest of the procedure, going from this meeting to a published volume. I'd like to thank Lois Reynolds and Caroline Overy for walking around so much with the microphones today. And, of course, the Wellcome Trust because they fund our work. We are also very grateful to the Wellcome Trust for allowing us to meet here in their headquarters, and for funding this 'Witness Seminar' project. I'd particularly like to thank Catherine for her excellent chairing; getting us to a glass of wine absolutely on time, but very relevant and pertinent questions throughout. Thank you so much, Catherine. Thank you. [Applause]

Peckham: Thank you all very much. I really enjoyed it.

Appendix 1

Table of British Cohort Studies

National Survey of Health & Development (NSHD)	1946	This MRC survey collected data from birth of 5362 singleton babies born to married parents during one week in March in 1946. This was a socially stratified sample taken from initial maternity survey of 13 687 births recorded in England, Scotland and Wales during that week. Since 1946 the participants have been studied 22 times with a change in focus over the years. In childhood the emphasis was on the investigation of the effects of the home and school environment on physical and mental development and educational attainment; during adulthood, this emphasis changed to study the relationship between childhood health and development and social circumstances and adult health and function. More recently, as the cohort reaches retirement, the research includes a study of the biological and social processes of ageing. See www.nshd.mrc.ac.uk/default.aspx (visited 23 January 2012).
National Child Development Study (NCDS)	1958	This study gathered data from almost 17 500 babies born in one week in March 1958 in England, Scotland and Wales. It was sponsored by the National Birthday Trust Fund, and was designed to examine the social and obstetric factors associated with stillbirth and death in early infancy among the children born in Great Britain. Since 1958, there have to date been eight further sweeps of the members of the birth cohort to monitor their physical, educational, social and economic development. See www.cls.ioe.ac.uk/page.aspx?&sitesectionid=724&sitesectiontitle=National+Child+Development+Study (visited 21 March 2012).
1970 British Cohort Study (BCS70)	1970	Originally called the British Births Survey (BBS), this study was sponsored by the National Birthday Trust Fund in association with the Royal College of Obstetricians and Gynaecologists. Information was collected about the births and families of just under 17 200 babies born in England, Scotland, Wales and Northern Ireland in a week in April 1970. Since then there have been seven follow-ups to gather information from the whole cohort with the emphasis of the study expanding from a strictly medical focus at birth, to include physical, educational and social development and, more recently, to include economic development and other wider factors. See www.cls.ioe.ac.uk/page.aspx?&sitesectionid=795&sitesectiontitle=Welcome+to+the+1970+British+Cohort+Study (visited 21 March 2012).

Avon Longitudinal Study of Parents and Children (ALSPAC)	1991–2	Originally called The Avon Longitudinal Study of Pregnancy and Childhood and also known as Children of the 90s, ALSPAC is a long-term health research project, in the former county of Avon, which has followed more than 14 000 children due between April 1991 and December 1992, from their mothers' pregnancies onwards. Data is collected on health, lifestyle and environment as well as biological samples of urine, blood and DNA. The vast amount of data has been used to establish genetic and environmental determinants of development and health. See www.bristol.ac.uk/alspac/ (visited 23 January 2012).
Millennium Cohort Study (MCS)	2000	Commissioned by the Economic and Social Research Council (ESRC), with funding supplemented by a consortium of government departments and the Wellcome Trust, this study follows the lives of around 19 000 children, selected through child benefit records, born in all four UK countries in 2000/1; it includes children from disadvantaged social circumstances and ethnic minorities. The study covers topics such as parenting, childcare, education, behaviour and cognitive development, health, social background and ethnicity. Surveys of cohort members were carried out at age nine months, three, five and seven years; the next is scheduled for 2012. See http://cls.nemisys2.uk.com/page.aspx?&sitesectionid =851&sitesectiontitle=Welcome+to+the+Millennium+Cohort +Study (visited 26 January 2012).
Birth Cohort Study	2012	This study, funded by the Department of Business Innovation and Skills (BIS), the Economic and Social Research Council (ESRC) and the MRC, will be the largest UK-wide study of babies and young children, and will follow over 90 000 children and their families from pregnancy through to the early years. It has been designed to reflect the diversity of ethnic identity and social backgrounds and will address important issues for children's health and well-being: for example the effects of parenting styles, the influence of eating and physical activity behaviours, and the effects of exposure to a range of environmental pollutants during early infancy. See, www.esrc. ac.uk/news-and-events/press-releases/14822/24-million-boost-to-uks-biggest-study-of-babies-and-young-children.aspx (visited 23 January 2012).

Appendix 2

A summary timeline of the origins and development of the Avon Longitudinal Study of Parents and Children (ALSPAC) for the Witness Seminar 24 May 2011.[161]

1978	Jean Golding (JG) commissioned by DoH to design a 1982 UK national birth cohort study
1979	National birth cohort for 1982 not funded
1985	JG asked by the World Health Organization to design a European set of cohort studies (becomes ELSPAC)
1985	Start of planning and piloting for ALSPAC, one of the European cohorts
1988	JG enlists Marcus Pembrey to lead the genetic aspects
1988	Pilot studies for collecting and storing cord blood and placentas
1989	ALSPAC Scientific Steering Committee formed
1990	Formation of ALSPAC Ethics and Law Committee
1990	Start of enrolment of pregnant women and questionnaires distributed to parents
1990	Start of storage of maternal blood and urine collected in pregnancy
1991	Start of collection of cord blood samples and placentas
1991	December – study goes into the red
1992	First of six monthly examinations of the 10 per cent sample 'Children in Focus'
1993	The last eligible babies born
1994	Blood for DNA taken at the 'Children in Focus' clinic
1995	Genetic Advisory Committee formed

---

[161] Adapted from a timeline supplied by Professor Jean Golding and distributed at the Witness Seminar.

1996	Strategic MRC award for DNA-banking
1996	Questionnaire administration to study children
1997	Completion of 'Children in Focus' study
1997	Questionnaires to local teachers initiated
1998	Start of clinical examination and blood for DNA from all study children
1998	First genetics paper (Dunger *et al.* (1998)) published
2000	DNA bank for 11 000 children and 10 000 mothers completed (Jones *et al.* (2000))
2000	Start of nine-year annual examination and blood samples taken for cell lines
2001	Wellcome Trust, MRC, University of Bristol, start (partial) core funding, including future generation of EBV-transformed cell lines from child and parent samples

Appendix 3

Funding contributions towards the Children in Focus Study[162]

III.4   FUNDING SECURED

Contributions towards the Children in Focus study have been received from the following:

FUNDER		PROJECT
1.	Medical Research Council	Vision screening (up to age 3) Parenting assessment (at 12 mo) Air pollution (NO_2) Short-term memory (at 5 years) Genetics of fetal growth
2.	South West Regional Health Authority	Infant anaemia Vision screening Dental amalgam Helicobacter infection
3.	Cow and Gate	Dietary diaries Infant anaemia
4.	Meat and Livestock Commission	Infant anaemia
5.	British Gas	Air pollution
6.	Milupa	4-month diet Vision
7.	Department of Health	Day-care
8.	Clothworkers Guild	Glue ear
9.	British Heart Foundation	Fingerprints Placental studies Blood pressure
10.	Northern Region Research and Development Directorate	Cholesterol Blood pressure Diet
11.	National Institutes of Health, U.S.A.	Hearing (at 31 mo)
12.	Department of the Environment	Lead
13.	Smith's Charities	Glue ear
14.	Wellcome Trust	Genetics of growth in first 2 years
15.	Remedi	Speech and language 2½ years
16.	MAFF	Food allergy
17.	Special Trustees	Factor V Leiden and pre-eclampsia

Contributions in kind from:

Child Growth Foundation, Oral B, Britmax, Pharmacia, Bedfont, Johnson & Johnson Medical Ltd., Scotia Pharmaceuticals.

---

[162] *Children in Focus. Development and Progress,* 3rd edition, June 1997: 89–90. Provided by Mrs Yasmin Iles-Caven, and reproduced by permission of Professor Jean Golding.

Appendix 4

Table of approximate numbers of grants submitted between 1989 and December 2005[163]

Funder type	Awarded	Failed
Wellcome Trust	41	47
Research councils	23	68
Other charities	60	160
Health authorities	16	39
Commercial sector applications	32	10
UK government	40	58
US government	20	35
EU	3	16
Total	235	433 (at least)

[163] Table supplied by Mrs Iles-Caven. E-mail to Ms Caroline Overy, 19 September 2011.

Appendix 5

Extract from the Human Fertilisation and Embryology Bill, House of Lords, 1990[164]

The Lord Chancellor: ... As I indicated in the earlier debate, in many cases where infertility treatment is not involved, the information about a child's father on the birth record may not reflect the true genetic position. That can arise for a number of reasons; for example, the mother may not know who the child's father is because she was having sexual intercourse with another man as well as her husband at the relevant time. After all, the birth register is a record and not a legal statement about the reality of who the child's father is. The noble Lady, Lady Saltoun, said that a doctor may ask what one's father died of. There is a chance that if one proceeds on the basis of what is shown on the birth certificate one may not give the correct answer. That is one of the problems.

In that connection, the noble Viscount, Lord Craigavon, mentioned the figure of 5 per cent. I have had an opportunity to look at that matter more closely. It is misleading to believe that at present the information on a birth certificate necessarily contains the full facts about the birth of a child. Members of the Committee will remember the surprise which greeted the reply made by my noble friend Lady Hooper on Second Reading. She indicated that clinical geneticists tell us that about one in 20 of today's population has a father other than the one named on the birth certificate. "Wrong paternity", if I may describe it as such, is an important matter to such medical specialists because, for reasons that have been outlined, they must take account of it in their clinical practice.

I am not aware of any published research reports from which one can derive with certainty an estimate of the prevalence of this state of affairs. But, in an article published in *Nature* on 26th October 1989, mention was made of a figure of 10 per cent. I have discussed the question with Professor Marcus Pembery [sic], Professor of Paediatric Genetics at the Institute of Child Health in London. From his experience, he believes that 10 per cent may be a somewhat high estimate. In his view, research studies where wrong paternity is an incidental

---

[164] Human Fertilisation and Embryology Bill [H.L.] Lords Hansard; Column 1317, HL Deb 13 February 1990 vol 515 c1317–c1318. Contains Parliamentary information licensed under the Open Parliament Licence v1.0; http://www.parliament.uk/site-information/copyright/open-parliament-licence/

finding, and clinical experience of clinical geneticists up and down the country each of whom has a service covering a wide geographical area, point to a prevalence of at least 5 per cent.

The importance of the matter is stressed in at least one text book and it takes up the point that I made in relation to the comment of the noble Lady, Lady Saltoun. An article written by Peter Harper, appearing on page 7 of *Practical Genetic Counselling*, 3rd edition, published in 1988, states: 'Illegitimacy must be borne in mind, especially in a puzzling situation. A family doctor or nurse may well, particularly in a small community, be able to clarify this possibility. Illegitimacy is not of course the problem, but mistaken paternity. New and definitive tests of paternity based on DNA will help to resolve those problems more easily, but may equally produce new difficulties by the more frequent detection of unsuspected non-paternity'. '1318 A person investigating the incidence of a genetic disease may have genetic DNA records of more than one generation. It is possible for those who are skilled in the science to tell in some instances whether the genetic quality of a child is compatible with the parents. The result is that sometimes, quite incidentally and not as part of any deliberate study, that is apparent. Of course, if the treatment or diagnosis is based on the birth certificate, as is obvious, mistakes can be made. The science of genealogy, in so far as it rests on birth certificates, is not on completely secure foundations. Nevertheless, it is still an important subject.

The birth certificate as such is not necessarily a correct record of the situation. Of course, the birth certificate has always to be understood in the light of the existing law. The noble Lord, Lord Henderson of Brompton, referred to the kindly presumption of paternity, which exists, and has existed for many years, in respect of a child born in wedlock.

Appendix 6

Letter of instructions for the ALSPAC Air Study[165]

The Avon Longitudinal Study of Pregnancy and Childhood
(ALSPAC)

Children of the Nineties
Institute of Child Health
University of Bristol
24 Tyndall Avenue
Bristol, BS2 8BJ
Tel: Hotline (0272) 256260

Thursday 19th November 1992

Dear Mother

Air Study

We are enclosing the tubes for air measurement as promised. Please put them in position this weekend. The instructions are as follows:

Indoor Tube with RED and WHITE caps

1.   The tube is to be stuck in the room where the baby normally sleeps. (Good surfaces for attaching the tubes include painted surfaces such as door frames).

2.   The position of the tube should be at about adult head height, where children and pets cannot reach it.
    The tube should NOT be stuck directly above the baby's cot in case the tube falls off the wall into the cot.

3.   Gently remove the **WHITE** cap from the end of the tube. **Please do not remove the red cap.**

4.   Peel off the paper from the blue sticky strip. Press it lengthwise on the tube but <u>do not cover the number.</u>

5.   **With the open end downwards,** press the tube onto the wall (or door frame) so it sticks.

6.   Write on the enclosed RECORDING SHEET, the date and time when the tube was put in position. Keep this sheet and the white cap in a safe place. The cap will be used later to reseal the tube.

Outdoor Tube with BLUE and WHITE Caps

1.   The tube must be stuck on the <u>outside</u> of the window or window-frame on the side of the house or flat which faces the street.

2.   Gently remove the **WHITE** cap from the end of the tube. **Please do not remove the blue cap.**

3.   Peel off the second sticky strip. Press it lengthwise onto the tube, but <u>do not cover the number.</u>

Steering Committee:
Professor J. D. Baum, Professor G. M. Stirrat,
Professor M. Pembrey, Professor C. Peckham, Professor J. Golding,
Professor M. Rutter, Professor J. Berry, Dr. C. Pennock, Dr. J. I. Pollock.

Recycled Paper

---

[165] Provided by Mrs Ruth Bowles and reproduced with permission of Professor Jean Golding.

4

4.   **With the open end downwards**, press the tube onto the outside of the window or window-frame so it sticks.

5.   Write on the enclosed RECORDING SHEET the date and time when the tube was put in position. Keep this sheet and the WHITE cap in a safe place. As with the other tube, the cap will be used later to reseal the tube.

We will send you further instructions for returning the tubes to us in 2 weeks.

This study will be unique in Avon in looking at the effect of outdoor pollution on indoor air quality. We would be most grateful for your help and cooperation.

With best wishes,

Yours sincerely,

Jean Golding

Professor Jean Golding.

Appendix 7

The Teenage Advisory Panel[166]

The first meeting of the ALSPAC Teenage Advisory Panel (TAP) was in July 2006, but this had been preceded for some years by ALSPAC children's Focus Groups. These had been set up and run by the ALSPAC Family Liaison Team and were half-day discussion forums, three to four times per year, comprising different ALSPAC study children each time, that endeavoured to elicit the children's opinions on a range of subjects.

TAP was initiated by Lynn Molloy, Executive Director of ALSPAC, the Family Liaison Team and other members of ALSPAC staff. Initially 25 young study participants were recruited from over 200 applicants who had submitted their *curricula vitarum* and their reasons for wanting to take part. The panel were chosen to be representative of the cohort by age, gender and social class. They met monthly until they were 16 and then once every two months to accommodate their busy lives. They also attended several away days and a residential weekend plus various training programmes in order to increase their understanding and effectiveness. In 2007 TAP elected its own chair and secretary who took over from ALSPAC staff who had been fulfilling these functions. In this year a dedicated participation worker was appointed to work closely with the panel. By 2008 the panel had expanded to 40 study participants.

Members of the ALSPAC Ethics and Law Committee attended TAP at the beginning of 2007 to discuss with the young people how they could appropriately become involved with ALSPAC's ethical process. It was decided that two representatives from TAP would attend the committee whenever possible.

From October 2007, when the first TAP representative attended the ALSPAC Ethics and Law Committee, until December 2009, TAP representatives attended the committee sporadically (although they were invited to every meeting). More frequent representation from TAP would have been useful as continuity is important in order to grasp the complexity of the ethical issues but it was known that these participants had very busy schedules and lunchtime

---

[166] This Appendix was written by Professor Gordon Stirrat. E-mail to Ms Caroline Overy, 13 December 2011.

meetings were difficult for them to attend. Nevertheless the contributions made by the representatives were considered extremely useful and frequently provided a perspective not necessarily obvious to the committee. On one occasion there was some reserved business on the agenda and, since the TAP representative was not a full member of the committee, he was informed beforehand that he would be asked to leave for this discussion. He, unfortunately, took this personally, and was annoyed but when it was explained that this was normal procedure in such committees, he accepted it. He was, in fact, a most valuable contributor to the meetings!

During 2009, it was decided that as the participants were reaching the age of 18, full committee membership for teenage participants would be appropriate. Three TAP representatives who had attended the committee, and were based locally, were elected to join the committee on the understanding that no more than two would attend each meeting. These representatives were considered full members of the committee and were treated in the same way as all the other committee members.

Key Achievements:

- Extensive collaboration with lead researchers to advise on content and delivery of questionnaires and other mailings.

- Instrumental in planning the décor and ambience for the two most recent clinics and introducing a 'Big Brother'-style room to enable participants attending the clinic to give their views of the study.

- Substantial ongoing input into the creation of an ALSPAC Facebook group – this method of communication is important for keeping in touch with the cohort.

- Involvement in the recruitment and interviewing of candidates for the posts of participation worker and the data linkage staff for a project funded by the Wellcome Trust.

- Attendance and then full membership of the ALSPAC Ethics and Law Committee meetings and representing the study at two ethics symposia.

References

Adams J, Bekhradnia B. (2004) *What future for dual support?* Report of Higher Education Policy Institute, page 19, www.hepi.ac.uk/466-1079/What-Future-for-Dual-Support-.html (visited 1 February 2012).

Advisory Board for the Research Councils (ABRC). (1987) *A Strategy for the Science Base;* a discussion document prepared for the Secretary of State for Education and Science by the Advisory Board for the Research Councils. London: HMSO.

Anon. (1989) Study on factors influencing child health. *Lancet* **334:** 518.

Bartington S E, Peckham C, Brown D, Joshi H, Dezateux C, Millennium Cohort Study Child Health Group. (2009) Feasibility of collecting oral fluid samples in the home setting to determine seroprevalence of infections in a large-scale cohort of preschool-aged children. *Epidemiology and Infection* **137:** 211–18.

Birdsong W M. (1998) The placenta and cultural values. *Western Medical Journal,* **168:** 190–2.

British Paediatric Association. Working Party on Ethics of Research in Children. (1980) Guidelines to aid ethical committees considering research involving children. *Archives of Disease in Childhood* **55:** 75–7.

British Paediatric Association. (1992) *Guidelines for the Ethical Conduct of Medical Research Involving Children* prepared by the Ethics Advisory Committee. London: British Paediatric Association.

Chadeau-Hyam M, Athersuch T J, Keun H C, De Iorio M, Ebbels T M, Jenab M, Sacerdote C, Bruce S J, Holmes E, Vineis P. (2011) Meeting-in-the-middle using metabolic profiling – a strategy for the identification of intermediate biomarkers in cohort studies. *Biomarkers* **16:** 83–8.

Chomczynski P, Sacchi N. (1987) Single-step method of RNA isolation by acid guanidinium thiocyanate-phenol-chloroform extraction. *Analytical Biochemistry* **162:** 156–9; doi: dx.doi.org/10.1016/0003-2697(87)90021-2

Chomczynski P, Sacchi N. (2006) The single-step method of RNA isolation by acid guanidinium thiocyanate-phenol-chloroform extraction: twenty-something years on. *Nature Protocols* **1:** 581–5; doi:10.1038/nprot.2006.83

Crowther S M, Reynolds L A, Tansey E M. (eds) (2009) *History of Dialysis in the UK: c.1950–1980.* Wellcome Witnesses to Twentieth Century Medicine, volume 37. London: The Wellcome Trust Centre for the History of Medicine at UCL; www.history.qmul.ac.uk/research/modbiomed/Publications/wit_vols/44867.pdf (visited 6 February 2012).

Department of Health. (1989) *On the State of the Public Health for the Year 1988: The annual report of the Chief Medical Officer.* London: HMSO.

Donald A E, Charakida M, Falaschetti E, Lawlor D A, Halcox J P, Golding J, Hingorani A D, Davey Smith G, Deanfield J E. (2010) Determinants of vascular phenotype in a large childhood population: the Avon Longitudinal Study of Parents and Children (ALSPAC). *European Heart Journal* **31:** 1502–10.

Doxiadis S. (ed.) (1989) *Early Influences Shaping the Individual.* NATO ASI Series A: Life Sciences, vol. 160. New York, NY: Plenum Press.

Dragonas T, Thorpe K, Golding J. (1992) Transition to fatherhood: a cross-cultural comparison. *Journal of Psychosomatic Obstetrics and Gynaecology* **13:** 1–19.

Dunger D B, Ong K K, Huxtable S J, Sherriff A, Woods K A, Ahmed M L, Golding J, Pembrey M E, Ring S, Bennett S T, Todd J A. (1998) Association of the INS VNTR with size at birth. ALSPAC Study Team. Avon Longitudinal Study of Pregnancy and Childhood. *Nature Genetics* **19:** 98–100.

Elliott P, Peakman T C. (2008) The UK Biobank sample handling and storage protocol for the collection, processing and archiving of human blood and urine. *International Journal of Epidemiology* **37:** 234–44 ; doi: 10.1093/ije/dym276

Elliott J, Shepherd P. (2006) Cohort Profile: 1970 British Birth Cohort (BCS70). *International Journal of Epidemiology* **35:** 836–43; doi: 10.1093/ije/dyl174

Emond A M. (1987) *The Spleen in Sickle Cell Disease in Childhood.* MD Thesis, University of Cambridge.

Emond A M, Hawkins N, Pennock C, Golding J. (1996) Haemoglobin and ferritin concentrations in infants at 8 months of age. *Archives of Disease in Childhood* **74:** 36–9; doi:10.1136/adc.74.1.36

Emond A, Howat P, Evans J-A, Hunt L. (1997) The effects of housing on the health of preterm infants. *Paediatric and Perinatal Epidemiology* **11:** 228–39.

Eysenck H J, Eysenck S B S. (1975) *Manual of The Eysenck Personality Questionnaire.* London: Hodder & Stoughton.

Fergusson D M, Horwood L J, Shannon F T, Lawton J M. (1989) The Christchurch Child Development Study: a review of epidemiological findings. *Paediatric and Perinatal Epidemiology* **3:** 302–25.

Fletcher L, Porter R. (1997) *A Quest for the Code of Life: Genome analysis at the Wellcome Trust Genome Campus.* London: Wellcome Trust.

Golding J. (1989a) European longitudinal study of pregnancy and childhood. *Paediatric and Perinatal Epidemiology* **3:** 460–9.

Golding J. (1989b) Illegitimate births: Do they suffer in the long-term? In Doxiadis S. (ed.) *Early Influences Shaping the Individual.* NATO ASI Series A: Life Sciences, vol. 160. New York, NY: Plenum Press: 111–121.

Golding J. (2009) The overall placing and management structure of a longitudinal birth cohort. *Paediatric and Perinatal Epidemiology* **23** (Suppl. 1): 23–30.

Golding J, Pembrey M, Jones R. (2001) ALSPAC – the Avon Longitudinal Study of Parents and Children. I. Study methodology. *Paediatric and Perinatal Epidemiology* **15:** 74–87.

Grant M. (ed.) (1985) *Alcohol Policies.* WHO Regional Publications, European Series, No 18. Copenhagen: World Health Organization Regional Office for Europe.

Hardy J, Singleton A. (2009) Genomewide association studies and human disease. *New England Journal of Medicine* **360:** 1759–68.

Harper P S, Reynolds L A, Tansey E M. (eds) (2010) *Clinical Genetics in Britain: Origins and development.* Wellcome Witnesses to Twentieth Century Medicine, volume 39. London Wellcome Trust Centre for the History of Medicine at UCL; www.history.qmul.ac.uk/research/modbiomed/wellcome_witnesses/volume39/index.html (visited 14 February 2012).

Hazelgrove J. (2001) Nuremberg Code. In Lock S, Last J M, Dunea G. (eds) *The Oxford Illustrated Companion to Medicine.* Oxford: Oxford University Press, 559–61.

House of Lords. (1990) Human Fertilisation and Embryology Bill [H.L.] Lords *Hansard;* Column 1317, HL Deb 13 February 1990, vol. 515 c1317–c1318.

Jones R W, Ring S, Tyfield L, Hamvas R, Simmons H, Pembrey M, Golding J, the ALSPAC Study Team. (2000) A new human genetic resource: a DNA bank established as part of the Avon Longitudinal Study of Pregnancy and Childhood (ALSPAC). *European Journal of Human Genetics* **8**: 653–60.

Kingman J F C. (1980) *Mathematics of Genetic Diversity.* Philadelphia, PA: Society for Industrial and Applied Mathematics.

Kingman J F C. (1993) *Poisson Processes.* Oxford Studies in Probability 3. Oxford: Clarendon Press.

Kingman J F C, Taylor S J. (1966) *Introduction to Measure and Probability.* Cambridge: Cambridge University Press.

Kleinman J C, Pierre M B, Jr, Madans J H, Land G H, Schramm W F. (1988) The effects of maternal smoking on fetal and infant mortality. *American Journal of Epidemiology* **127**: 274–82.

Lander J, Hodgins M, Nazarali S, McTavish J, Ouellette J, Friesen E. (1996) Determinants of success and failure of EMLA. *Pain* **64**: 89–97.

Lock S, Last J M, Dunea G. (eds) (2001) *The Oxford Illustrated Companion to Medicine.* Oxford: Oxford University Press.

McIntosh I D. (1984) Smoking and pregnancy: II. Offspring risks. *Public Health Reviews* **12**: 29–63.

MacIntyre S, Sooman A. (1991) Non-paternity and prenatal genetic screening. *Lancet* **338**: 869–71.

Malcolm S, Clayton-Smith J, Nichols M, Robb S, Webb T, Armour J A L, Jeffreys A J, Pembrey M E. (1991) Uniparental paternal disomy in Angelman's syndrome. *Lancet* **337**: 694–7.

Mason J K, McCall Smith R A. (1989) *Law and Medical Ethics,* 2nd edn. London: Butterworth.

Medical Research Council. (1991) *The Ethical Conduct of Research on Children.* London: Medical Research Council.

Moise K J Jr. (2005) Umbilical cord stem cells. *Obstetrics and Gynecology* **106**: 1393–407.

Mumford S E. (1999a) Children of the 90s: ethical guidance for a longitudinal study. *Archives of Disease in Childhood. Fetal and Neonatal Edition* **81**: F146–51.

Mumford S E. (1999b) Children of the 90s II: challenges for the ethics and law committee. *Archives of Disease in Childhood. Fetal and Neonatal Edition* **81**: F228–31.

Nicholson R H. (ed.) (1986) *Medical Research with Children: Ethics, law, and practice: the report of an Institute of Medical Ethics working group on the ethics of clinical research investigations on children.* Oxford: Oxford University Press.

Ong K K L, Ahmed M L, Sherriff A M, Woods K A, Watts A, Golding J, the ALSPAC Study Team, Dunger D B. (1999) Cord blood leptin is associated with size at birth and predicts infancy weight gain in humans. *Journal of Clinical Endocrinology and Metabolism* **84**: 1145–8.

Owens M E, Todt E H. (1984) Pain in infancy: Neonatal reaction to a heel lance. *Pain* **20**: 77–86.

Pappworth M H. (1967) *Human Guinea Pigs: Experimentation on man.* London: Routledge and Kegan Paul.

Paternoster L, Lorentzon M, Vandenput L, Karlsson M K, Ljunggren Ö, Kindmark A, Mellstrom D, Kemp J P, Jarett C E, Holly J M P, Sayers A, St Pourcain B, Timpson N J, Deloukas P, Davey Smith G, Ring S M, Evans D M, Tobias J H, Ohlsson C. (2010) Genome-wide association meta-analysis of cortical bone mineral density unravels allelic heterogeneity at the RANKL locus and potential pleiotropic effects on bone. *PLoS Genetics* **6**: e1001217.

Peckham C S. (1972) Clinical and laboratory study of children exposed *in utero* to maternal rubella. *Archives of Disease in Childhood* **47**: 571–7.

Peckham C S. (1973) A national study of child development (NCDS 1958 cohort). Preliminary findings in a national sample of 11-year-old children. *Proceedings of the Royal Society of Medicine.* **66**: 701–3.

Peckham C S, Coleman J C, Hurley R, Chin K S, Henderson K, Preece P M. (1983) Cytomegalovirus in pregnancy: preliminary findings from a prospective study. *Lancet* **321:** 1352–5.

Peckham C S, Senturia Y D, Ades A E, Newell M L, Giaquinto C, De Rossi A, Chieco-Bianchi L, Zacchello F, Mok J Y Q, Hague R, Grosch-Worner I, Koch S, Canosa C A, Omenaca Teres F, Garcia Rodriguez M C, Scherpbier H J, Bohlin A B, De Maria A, Gotta C, Terragna A, for the European Collaborative Study. (1988) Mother-to-child transmission of HIV infection. *Lancet* **322:** 1039–43.

Pembrey M. (1989) Advances in genetic prediction and diagnosis. In Doxiadis S. (ed.) *Early Influences Shaping the Individual.* NATO ASI Series A: Life Sciences, vol. 160. New York, NY: Plenum Press: 23–35.

Pembrey M E. (1990) Cohort of genes. *Nature* **348:** 280.

Pembrey M E, Bygren L O, Kaati G, Edvinsson S, Northstone K, Sjöström M, Golding J, the ALSPAC Study Team. (2006) Sex-specific, male-line transgenerational responses in humans. *European Journal of Human Genetics* **14:** 159–66.

Power C, Elliott J. (2006) Cohort profile: 1958 British Cohort Study. *International Journal of Epidemiology* **35:** 34–41.

Preece A W, Kaune W T, Grainger P, Golding J. (1999) Assessment of human exposure to magnetic fields produced by domestic appliances. *Radiation Protection Dosimetry* **83:** 21–7.

Puissant C, Houdebine L M. (1990) An improvement of the single-step method of RNA isolation by acid guanidinium thiocyanate-phenol-chloroform extraction. *Biotechniques* **8:** 148–9.

Relton C L, Davey Smith G. (2010) Epigenetic epidemiology of common complex disease: prospects for prediction, prevention and treatment. *PLoS Medicine* **7:** e1000356.

Relton C L, Groom A, St Pourcain B, Sayers A E, Swan D C, Embleton N D, Pearce M S, Ring S M, Northstone K, Tobias J H, Trakalo J, Ness A R, Shaheen S O, Davey Smith G. (2012) DNA methylation patterns in cord blood DNA and body size in childhood. *PLoS ONE* **7:** e31821; doi:10.1371/journal.pone.0031821

Reynolds L A, Tansey E M. (eds) (2007) *Medical Ethics Education in Britain, 1963–93.* Wellcome Witnesses to Twentieth Century Medicine, volume 31. London: Wellcome Trust Centre for the History of Medicine at UCL. Freely available online at www.history.qmul.ac.uk/research/modbiomed/ wellcome_witnesses/ volume31/index.html (visited 6 February 2012).

Riis P. (2001) Declaration of Helsinki. In Lock S, Last J M, Dunea G. (eds) *The Oxford Illustrated Companion to Medicine,* 3rd edn. Oxford: Oxford University Press, 373–4.

Rogers T L, Ostrow C L. (2004) The use of EMLA cream to decrease venipuncture pain in children. *Journal of Pediatric Nursing* **19**: 33–9.

Royal College of Physicians. (1967) *Supervision of the Ethics of Clinical Research Investigations in Institutions.* London: Royal College of Physicians of London.

Royal College of Physicians. (1990) *Research Involving Patients.* London: Royal College of Physicians of London.

Sargent I L, Redman C W, Stirrat G M. (1982) Maternal cell-mediated immunity in normal and pre-eclamptic pregnancy. *Clinical & Experimental Immunology* **50**: 601–9.

Sawyer P. (2008) NHS hospital sells placentas for cosmetic use. *The Telegraph* (17 May) www.telegraph.co.uk/news/1973229/NHS-hospital-sells-placentas-for-cosmetic-use.html (visited 6 February 2012).

Shah V, Ohlsson A. (2007) Venepuncture versus heel lance for blood sampling in term neonates. *Cochrane Database of Systematic Reviews* **4**: CD001452.

Shah V S, Taddio A, Bennett S, Speidel B D. (1997) Neonatal pain response to heel stick vs venepuncture for routine blood sampling. *Archives of Disease in Childhood* **77**: F143–4.

Sherriff A, Farrow A, Golding J, the ALSPAC Study Team, Henderson J. (2005) Frequent use of chemical household products is associated with persistent wheezing in pre-school age children. *Thorax* **60**: 45–9.

Simpson W J. (1957) A preliminary report on cigarette smoking and the incidence of prematurity. *American Journal of Obstetrics and Gynecology* **73**: 808–15.

Slater R, Cantarella A, Gallella S, Worley A, Boyd S, Meek J, Fitzgerald M. (2006) Cortical pain responses in human infants. *Journal of Neuroscience* **26:** 3662–6.

Sunderland C A, Naiem M, Mason D Y, Redman C W G, Stirrat G M. (1981) The expression of major histocompatibility antigens by human chorionic villi. *Journal of Reproductive Immunology* **3:** 323–31.

Thorpe K J, Dragonas T, Golding J. (1992a) The effects of psychosocial factors on the emotional well-being of women during pregnancy: A cross-cultural study of Britain and Greece. *Journal of Reproductive and Infant Psychology* **10:** 191–204; doi: 10.1080/02646839208403953

Thorpe K J, Dragonas T, Golding J. (1992b) The effects of psychosocial factors on the mother's emotional well-being during early parenthood: A cross-cultural study of Britain and Greece. *Journal of Reproductive and Infant Psychology* **10:** 205–17; doi: 10.1080/02646839208403954

US, National Commission for the Protection of Human Subjects of Biomedical and Behavioral Research. (1978) *The Belmont Report: Ethical principles and guidelines for the protection of human subjects of research.* Washington: US Government Print Office.

Wellcome Trust, Portfolio Review. (2010) Human genetics research timeline. *Human Genetics 1990–2009.* London: The Wellcome Trust, 73–80; www.wellcome.ac.uk/stellent/groups/corporatesite/@policy_communications/documents/web_document/wtx063661.pdf (visited 6 February 2012).

Welshman J. (2012) Time, money and social science: the British Birth Cohort Surveys of 1946 and 1958. *Social History of Medicine* **25:** 175–92.

Biographical notes[*]

Professor (John) David Baum
MD FRCP FRCPH FRCPE
FMedSci (1940–1999) was
lecturer, and then clinical reader
in paediatrics at Oxford University
from 1972, and in 1977 was
elected to a professorial fellowship
at St Catherine's College. He was
appointed professor of child health
at the University of Bristol in 1985
and from 1988 was a founding
director of the Institute of Child
Health (Bristol). He was President
of the Royal College of Paediatrics
and Child Health (1997–99).

Miss Karen Birmingham
SRN RMN (b. 1955) is currently
the research ethics manager
and ethics archive manager for
the Avon Study of Parents and
Children (ALSPAC). She trained
as a general and psychiatric nurse
at the London Hospital before
obtaining a diploma in psychosocial
and family-centred nursing at the
Cassel Hospital, Richmond, Surrey.
She worked clinically, mostly in
psychiatry, before having two years
at home as a full-time mother.
She joined the Department (later
the Institute) of Child Health,
Bristol, in 1988 when ALSPAC

was being planned and piloted.
She also worked with the Institute's
Respiratory Research Group for
several years. She diverted to
Pennsylvania for a year when she
was awarded a scholarship (Quaker
Studies & Social Change) but
returned to ALSPAC in 1995 to
supervise data abstraction from
medical records and other ALSPAC
sub-studies. She took over as the
secretary of the ALSPAC Ethics
and Law Committee in 1999.
She has recently been awarded
a visiting research post with the
Swiss Brocher Foundation to write
a monograph describing the work
of the Ethics and Law Committee
during its first 16 years.

Mrs Ruth Bowles
RGN BSc (b. 1960) qualified as
a state registered nurse at Royal
United Hospital, Bath, in 1982
and specialized in intensive care
nursing following additional studies
at the Bristol Royal Infirmary
in 1985. After a brief period as
sister in the coronary care and
intensive care unit at Weston
General Hospital 1987–88 was
senior sister in Cardiac Intensive
Care Unit, Bristol Royal Infirmary
(1988–2010). She completed

[*] Contributors are asked to supply details; other entries are compiled from conventional
biographical sources.

a BSc (Hons) in information technology and computing with the Open University (2008) and is currently heading the cardiac research nursing team at University Hospitals Bristol working on a portfolio of local, national and international cardiology and cardiac surgery interventional and observational trials. She has been a study participant since 1991 and a study mother member of the ALSPAC Law and Ethics Committee since 2001.

Sir Iain Chalmers
Kt FRCP FRGOG FFPH FMedSci (b. 1943) has been editor of the award-winning James Lind Library since 2003. He was director of the National Perinatal Epidemiology Unit, Oxford, from 1978 to 1992, and director of the UK Cochrane Centre in Oxford from 1992 to 2002.

Dr Ian A F Lister Cheese
MA PhD FRCP FRCPH (b.1936) read natural sciences followed by training in research under Walter Morgan. He trained in medicine, qualifying in 1966. Following posts as medical registrar to Sir George Pickering and Paul Beeson at the Radcliffe Infirmary, he entered general practice in Wantage, Oxfordshire. There he became a tutor in general practice, a trainer in the vocational training scheme

and served in NHS management in Oxfordshire. In 1984 he joined the senior civil service with appointments in the Department of Health and the Department of Education. His posts included responsibilities for the fitness of teachers, hospital services for children and for genetics services. He was secretary to the Standing Medical Advisory Committee and to the Gene Therapy Advisory Committee. He also served on the RCP Clinical Genetics Committee and committees of the BPA and subsequently of the RCPCH, and a number of MRC committees. Following notional retirement in 1996 he became an adviser to the Department of Health on matters relating to clinical governance and the working of the Abortion Act, has undertaken policy work for the RCP, the Academy of Medical Royal Colleges, and the National Director for Health and Work. He was a member of the editorial board that prepared the first edition of the new formulary, *Medicines for Children*. He also served as trustee to voluntary bodies concerned with the support of disabled children and their families.

Professor George Davey Smith
MA MSc MD FFPHM DSc, FRCP FMedSci (b. 1959) has been professor of clinical epidemiology at the University of Bristol since

1994. He is currently scientific director of the Avon Longitudinal Study of Parents and Children (ALSPAC) and director of the MRC Centre for Causal Analyses in Translational Epidemiology (CAiTE). He previously held appointments at the University of Cardiff, MRC Epidemiology Unit, South Wales, University College London, London School of Hygiene and Tropical Medicine and Glasgow University.

Professor Alan Emond
MA MD FRCP FRCPCH FHEA (b. 1953) is a clinical academic paediatrician. He graduated from Cambridge University in 1977 and, since training in internal medicine and paediatrics in the UK, Jamaica and Australia, he has been working in Bristol since 1985. He is professor of child health at the University of Bristol, head of the Centre for Child and Adolescent Health in Bristol and consultant paediatrician at North Bristol Trust and University Hospitals Bristol Trust. His clinical background is in general and community paediatrics, with over 30 years' experience of children's medicine and child public health. His research experience is in epidemiology and health service evaluation, including work on ALSPAC, and in clinical trials. He is currently chair of the British Paediatric Surveillance Unit. He

has published widely on child growth and development, and has advised the English government on policy for children. He is an experienced educator, with a special interest in inter-professional teaching and learning. From 2005–09, he was chair of the British Association of Community Child Health (BACCH), the national organization for community paediatricians in the UK. In 2003 he set up the Centre for Child and Adolescent Health in a joint initiative between the University of Bristol and the University of the West of England, creating a multi-disciplinary academic group undertaking research and teaching in community child health.

Professor Jean Golding
OBE, MA, PhD, DSc, FSS, MRCPCH, FMedSci (b. 1939) graduated in mathematics at Oxford in 1961. A career break for child care was followed by employment 1966–8 by the team analysing data from the 1958 Birth Survey followed by a research fellowship at the Galton Laboratory, department of human genetics and biometry to continue the analysis (1968–1971). Employment at Oxford University in Richard Doll's department of the Regius Professor of Medicine, and then the National Perinatal Epidemiology Unit was

then followed by a move to the University of Bristol in 1980, to the department of child health. She won a Wellcome senior lecturership in 1982, became a reader in 1988 and was appointed to a chair in 1992. She founded the international journal *Paediatric and Perinatal Epidemiology* in 1987 and continued as its editor-in-chief until 2012. She assisted in the design and analysis of birth surveys in Greece (1983) and Jamaica (1986), before creating the design and development of the ELSPAC and ALSPAC pre-birth cohorts; she continued as scientific and executive director of ALSPAC until the end of 2005. She is now emeritus professor of paediatric and perinatal epidemiology at the University of Bristol where she is still research-active. She was awarded an OBE for services to medical science in the New Year's honours list of 2012.

Professor David Gordon

FRCP FMedSci (b. 1947) is a general physician. He began his academic career in the medical unit at St Mary's Hospital Medical School. In a prolonged break from his conventional academic medical career he was a member of the staff of the Wellcome Trust, London, responsible for support of biological and medical research across a wide range of subjects, and for the career development of clinical and basic biomedical scientists. He worked at the University of Manchester (1999–2007), most of that time as dean of the medical faculty. He was chair of the Council of Heads of Medical Schools and is also the president of the Association of Medical Schools in Europe. He has been visiting professor at the University of Copenhagen since 2007, in the offices of the World Federation for Medical Education.

Mrs Yasmin Iles-Caven

Dip (Management Studies) (b. 1962) started working for Jean Golding in 1981 after completing her A levels, as a clerical assistant. From 1982 to 1999 she worked as Jean's personal assistant, and was responsible for supervising the secretarial team and typing mainly research grant applications with a growing responsibility for ALSPAC finances. In 1999 she was promoted to resources manager with responsibility for financial, personnel and physical resources for the Unit of Paediatric & Perinatal Epidemiology. In 2003, when the faculty underwent restructuring, she became departmental manager for ALSPAC. She acted as secretary to the ALSPAC Steering Committee (1999–2004) and to the University Management Committee. In 2006 ALSPAC was moved into the department of social medicine and her job title reverted back to resources manager. She continued in this capacity until December 2010 when she was made redundant. She is currently assisting Jean Golding with the archiving of pre-2005 ALSPAC documentation.

Dr Richard Wynn Jones

DPhil (b. 1943) after a career spent in molecular genetic research and as a chemical pathologist (MRC fellowship and honorary consultant in chemical pathology, MRC Unit of Molecular Haematology and John Radcliffe Hospital, Oxford, 1985–1992; senior lecturer and honorary consultant in chemical pathology, Institute of Child Health, University of London, 1993–2000), he helped to establish and develop the ALSPAC laboratory (senior research fellow, ALSPAC, University of Bristol, 2000–07). This laboratory is notable for its application of robotic automation to DNA-banking and of immortalized cell line production. Wider responsibilities included management of the study's banks of biological samples and liaising with research collaborators on the use of these resources.

Sir John Kingman

Kt FRS MA ScD (b. 1939) studied mathematics at the University of Cambridge. He was professor of mathematics and statistics the University of Sussex from 1966 to 1969 when he was appointed professor of mathematics at the University of Oxford, a post which he held until 1985, when he became vice-chancellor of the University of Bristol. From 2001 to 2006 he was the director of the Isaac Newton Institute for Mathematical Sciences, during which time he was the first N M Rothschild & Sons Professor of Mathematical Sciences. He was President of the Royal Statistical Society (1987–89), and of the London Mathematical Society (1990–92). He was knighted in 1985 for his work with the SERC of which he was chairman (1981–85).

Mrs Elizabeth Mumford

LLM (b. 1958) was educated at Stanford University, the University of Toronto and Queens' College Cambridge. She was a lecturer in law at King's College London and at Bristol University. She took an early 'retirement' in 2000 to embark on a late career as a mother but still lectures on a part-time basis in medical law at Bristol.

Professor Catherine Peckham
CBE MD FMedSci FRCP
FRCPCH FFPH FRCOG
FRCPath (b. 1937) is professor of
paediatric epidemiology and former
head of the Centre for Paediatric
Epidemiology and Biostatistics,
at the Institute of Child Health,
University College London. She has
worked on infections in pregnancy
and the consequences for the child
and has been closely involved in
national birth cohort studies. The
influence of biological, social and
environmental factors in early life
on later development has been a
central theme in her work. She has
published chapters and papers on
infections in pregnancy and early
childhood, the epidemiology of
common childhood conditions and
immunisation.

Professor Marcus Pembrey
MD FRCP FRCPCH FRCOG
FMedSci (b. 1943) trained in
medical genetics in Liverpool
(1969–71) and Guy's Hospital,
London (1973–78). In 1979 he
moved to the Institute of Child
Health, London, as head of the
Mothercare unit of paediatric
genetics where he led a team that
helped to introduce DNA testing
into clinical genetics in the 1980s.
He was also consultant clinical
geneticist at the Hospital for Sick
Children, Great Ormond Street,
London (1979–98) and consultant

adviser in genetics to the Chief
Medical Officer, Department
of Health (1989–98). He led
the genetic component of the
ALSPAC from 1988. After early
retirement from the ICH in 1998,
he continued as director of genetics
within ALSPAC, University of
Bristol, until 2006. He continues
to be visiting professor at the
University of Bristol.

Professor Brian Pickering
PhD DSc (b. 1936) is professor
emeritus in anatomy, University
of Bristol, and was deputy
vice-chancellor (1992–2001).
After a first degree in biological
chemistry, his research career
has been concerned with the
biosynthesis and physiology of
active polypeptides, principally the
neuroendocrine products of the
hypothalamus. After periods in
the Hormone Research Laboratory
of the University of California
(Berkeley), and NIMR, he was at
Bristol from 1965–2001, being
head of department of anatomy
(1978–1992) and dean of the
faculty of medicine (1985–87).
He was a founding member of the
British Neuroendocrine Group
(British Neuroendocrine Society
from 2001), serving as its first
secretary (de-facto chairman),
(1988–92). He served on AFRC/
BBSRC Animals Research Grants
Board (1988–94); chairman,

(1991–94), on Bristol & Weston Health Authority (1988–90) and as non-executive director, United Bristol Healthcare NHS Trust (1990–98).

Dr Jon Pollock

PhD (b. 1948) is a reader in epidemiology at the University of the West of England, Bristol. Originally trained as a zoologist and physical anthropologist in Edinburgh and UCL, he moved to Africa to teach postgraduate wildlife management and conservation to students at the University of Dar es Salaam in Tanzania. He spent two years managing a conservation centre for prosimians at Duke University, Durham, North Carolina before returning to Bristol University, where he was offered the opportunity by Professor Golding to work there on epidemiological studies of child development using national cohort study data. Drawn into the ALSPAC project by Professor Golding's imaginative enthusiasm, he played a small part in the early developmental planning stages of the project before focusing on evaluations of community-based children's services at home and abroad, with Professor Alan Emond. He left Bristol University, temporarily, to manage the new research department of the Royal College of Paediatrics and Child Health before returning to Bristol to direct the Department of Health-funded Research and Development Service Unit. He now works part-time for its successor, the Research Design Service.

Dr Susan Ring

PhD (b. 1967) is head of the ALSPAC Laboratories and a member of the current ALSPAC Executive Committee. Trained in genetics at Sheffield University and the Galton Laboratory, UCL, her early research interests included the genetics and biochemistry of blood group antigens and red cell membrane proteins. In 1996 she joined the molecular genetics department at Southmead Hospital, Bristol to establish the DNA bank for the ALSPAC study, moving to the University of Bristol in 2002 to continue working with ALSPAC and the 1958 birth cohort establishing cell line banks and developing the DNA and biobanks for both cohorts. She became head of the ALSPAC Laboratories in 2006.

Mrs Sue Sadler

BSc Cert Ed (b. 1943) was clinic manager at ALSPAC from 1992 to 2008. After training in Bristol she taught biology in secondary schools in the Bristol area. After the birth of her third child she was an antenatal teacher with the NCT for ten years. She served on Bristol

Community Health Council in the 1980s and with Maternity Links, which provided linkworker support for ethnic minority women. In September 1990 she joined ALSPAC working to recruit women from ethnic minorities, coding questionnaires, researching data on neonatal deaths, writing newsletters and liaising with hospitals over biological samples. She and Dr Jean Golding met with matrons of the maternity hospitals, whom she knew through NCT work, in order to obtain their support for the study. She organized the measuring of newborn study babies in hospital from September 1991 and the Children in Focus clinics from October 1992 for a subset of the children, followed by the Focus clinics for all participants from age seven. She managed these clinics until retirement in March 2008.

Professor Gordon Stirrat

MA MD FRCOG (b. 1940) is emeritus professor of obstetrics & gynaecology and research fellow in ethics in medicine in the University of Bristol. Having trained as an obstetrician and gynaecologist in Glasgow and London, he became clinical reader in the University of Oxford in 1975. He was appointed professor and head of department of obstetrics and gynaecology in the University of Bristol in 1982. While still holding this post he was appointed dean of the faculty of medicine (1991–93) and then pro-vice-chancellor (1993–97). He has been a Member of the Southwest Regional Health Authority (1984–90); the Bristol & Weston Health Authority (1990–92) and vice-chairman of Bristol & District Health Authority (1992–98). He served on the General Medical Council (1990–93) and was a member of the Central Research and Development Committee for the National Health Service (1990–94). He was chair of the Ethics Committees of the Royal College of Obstetricians & Gynaecologists (2001–2004) and of ALSPAC (2007–10). He is currently a member of the Governing Body of the Institute of Medical Ethics.

Professor Tilli Tansey

PhD PhD DSc HonFRCP FMedSci (b. 1953) is convenor of the History of Twentieth Century Medicine Group – known as the History of Modern Biomedicine Research Group from 2010 – and professor of the history of modern medical sciences at Queen Mary, University of London.

Dr Linda Tyfield

MSc PhD FRCPath (b. 1946) was a consultant clinical scientist and head of molecular genetics at Southmead Hospital, Bristol. After studying nutrition and biochemistry at the University of Toronto and Bristol University she specialized in the biochemical study of inherited metabolic disease at the clinical biochemistry department at Southmead Hospital. In 1988 she set up a molecular genetics unit there specializing in the genetic analysis of neurological and muscular diseases and later became head of the department of molecular genetics. Her research interests were in genetic variation in inherited metabolic disease, genetic variation within and between populations and genetic changes in neurological tumours. The extraction of DNA from samples collected for the ALSPAC cohort was originally developed and tested in her department. She has had many research collaborations with colleagues in Europe and North America. She was chairman of the Clinical Molecular Genetics Society from 2000 to 2004 and has served on many professional and government advisory committees.

Mr Mike Wall
DipLib MCLIP (b. 1965), a study father, has been head of information management at the University of Bristol since 2007. He has recently gained funding to scope and then deposit the ALSPAC archive at the University of Bristol Library.

Index: Subject

Index: Names

Biographical notes appear in bold

Key to cover photographs

Front cover, left to right
Professor Alan Emond
Mrs Elizabeth Mumford
Professor Marcus Pembrey
Professor Gordon Stirrat
Professor Jean Golding

Back cover, left to right
Mrs Yasmin Iles-Caven
Professor Brian Pickering
Mrs Sue Sadler
Dr Richard Jones
Mrs Ruth Bowles

Lightning Source UK Ltd.
Milton Keynes UK
UKOW020045300512

193579UK00003B/1/P